Clinical data mining
in an allied health organisation
A real world experience

Edited by Roslyn Giles, Irwin Epstein and Anne Vertigan

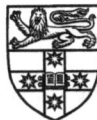

SYDNEY UNIVERSITY PRESS

Published 2011 by Sydney University Press
SYDNEY UNIVERSITY PRESS
University of Sydney Library
sydney.edu.au/sup

Sydney University Press
Fisher Library F03
University of Sydney NSW 2006 AUSTRALIA
Email: sup.info@sydney.edu.au

National Library of Australia Cataloguing-in-Publication entry

Title: Clinical data mining in an allied health organisation : a real
         world experience / edited by Roslyn Giles, Irwin Epstein
         and Anne Vertigan.
ISBN: 9781920899653 (pbk.)
Subjects: Data mining.
         Evidence-based medicine
         Medical care--Evaluation.
         Outcome assessment (Medical care)
Other Authors/Contributors:
         Giles, Roslyn.
         Epstein, Irwin.
         Vertigan, Anne.
Dewey Number:
         362.1

Cover design by Miguel Yamin, the University Publishing Service
Printed in Australia

Contents

Preface

Clinical data mining (CDM) is 'the practitioner's use of available agency data for practice-based research (PBR) purposes' (Epstein 2010). This collection represents the 'real world' product of several groups of allied health practitioner researchers conducting CDM studies of their own practice. For a practice-based research consultant like me, the process through which these studies were conceived, implemented and written about came as close to CDM heaven as it possibly could.

Hunter New England Health (HNE) is a thoroughly modern and forward-thinking healthcare service system. With a large hospital centre and smaller satellite settings, it is located in and around Newcastle, Australia, a place (like heaven) in which I never anticipated spending any time, let alone working. Once begun, however, working 'closely' via email with project leaders Ros Giles and Anne Vertigan, and annually and face-to-face with HNE's brilliant multidisciplinary staff, it became a joyfully productive transdisciplinary and transformational experience for me. I hope it was for them as well.

Let me say a few words about the organisational environment in which we worked. Not only does Newcastle possess a historic and present-day coal-mining culture like its original English namesake, but unlike its forebear, it boasts incredibly beautiful beaches and spectacular surf. With sunrise and the early morning tide, a more typically Aussie surfer scene emerges. But on any given night from shore can be seen the lights of countless tankers from coal-hungry industrial nations anchored far out at sea, patiently awaiting their fill.

And yet, the nearby Hunter Valley is justly famous for its superb and subtle wines, lovely vineyards and verdant landscape. This, dear reader, is no reminder of England's industrial north. Still, it was in New-castle, Australia, that I first heard social workers employ the expression 'working at the coalface' to refer to direct work with clients. So, in this Australian coal-mining town, CDM seemed to come naturally to HNE staff. For me, it brought me as close to working the multidisciplinary 'coalface' as ever before.

This data-mining exploration originated in 2005 with a CDM workshop co-conducted in Newcastle with Lynette Joubert from the University of Melbourne School of Social Work. The workshop was co-sponsored by HNE and the University of Newcastle Social Work program. The invitation for me to return and provide CDM consulta-tion to allied health professionals at HNE came from David Rhodes who was at the time HNE's Area Director of Allied Health. His ongoing support and his vision of how CDM could promote HNE's capacity for organisational and professional learning made this project possible.

The invitation was intriguing for several reasons. First, I had only recently been exposed to the concept of 'allied health'. Highly developed in Australia, it is rarely used in my experience in hospitals and health settings in the US. Siloed more than allied, health professions in the US are too often competitive and cut off from each other. Even multi-disciplinary team members know little of what other team members do. This became clear to me in several multidisciplinary CDM projects con-ducted at Mt Sinai Hospital in New York (Epstein & Blumenfield 2001).

Second, I had only just begun to appreciate the applicability of CDM as a practitioner-research strategy for health professions other than social work. Though I had recently co-edited with Dr Joubert a special issue of the *Journal of Social Work Research and Evaluation* de-voted to multidisciplinary CDM in Australian allied health (2005), I had never had the opportunity to implement CDM methodology in a single health setting as part of a larger organisational development and capacity-building effort.

What followed for me was a series of highly efficient, annual, one-day/one-night consulting trips to Newcastle coinciding with already scheduled annual consulting and lecturing visits to Melbourne. It didn't hurt that these 'one-nighters' included a stay in a lovely hotel, with an on-site, world-class restaurant serving local wines. After an exciting and exhausting day filled with back-to-back consultation sessions, working lunches, teleconferenced presentations to hospital and satellite staff, and meetings with the project leadership, I was each time rewarded with a superb dinner, dramatically overlooking the sea with a glass or two of superb local wines. I prefer the reds. (My only regret during those delicious solo dinners was that my wife wasn't there to share them with me. But no worries, I made up for that in February 2011 when after celebrating the University of Melbourne School of Social Work's 70th anniversary, I took her there to celebrate my 73rd birthday.)

Though I 'surfed' in and out of Newcastle on an annual basis, I was also aware that a solid support infrastructure of innumerable meetings, writing workshops, data-analysis consultations, leadership strategy sessions and paper re-writes took place throughout the years. These were provided by Anne Vertigan and Ros Giles. It was their co-captaining that kept this CDM 'tanker' on course, moving forward slowly but steadily. As we point out in our introductory essay, it wasn't all sun and surf. Some projects went under. Others kept bobbing up despite rough seas. Others seemed to experience smooth sailing from start to finish.

There were also positive 'spin-offs' that are not recorded in this book. For example, I well remember two radiation oncologists who after one of my large lectures stayed on for several working sessions with different allied health practitioner groups. The oncologists were interested in using their own available data to study their oncology practice but, in the process of learning about CDM, they were also learning about what various allied health professions actually did, thought about and conducted research on. Similarly I remember a pair of surgeons just 'sitting in' on one of the working sessions with speech pathologists focusing on 'thyroid voice'. The surgeons introduced themselves by saying that they only had five minutes to spare and were just wondering what we were up to. At the conclusion of our 45 minute session they were still there, talking about publication possibilities associated with the study.

Not part of the HNE project, but conducted in Newcastle, is a CDM study recently published describing a 'data-mining expedition' into 'single-session social work' in local hospital settings by Plath and Gibbons (2010) of the University of Newcastle. I like to think their study was inspired by Joubert's and my original CDM workshop. Maybe so, maybe not, but speaking about unanticipated outcomes, the irony did not escape me that, while personally suffering from spinal stenosis, I was editing and learning about my own treatment possibilities from a CDM article on low-back pain interventions with over 400 people like me by my HNE physical therapy colleagues.

Perhaps most personally gratifying about this project, however, was discovering how CDM methodology can be helpful in generating practice-based knowledge about health issues and interventions that I previously knew nothing about, working with professions other than my own and in contexts unlike any I had personally or professionally experienced. A case in point is the award-winning project on solastalgia among Australian farm families during periods of drought. A city boy, growing up in Brooklyn and spending 13 years teaching in Michigan, knows lots about longing for home but little about farming and drought, and its impact on mental health.

My first CDM article published a decade ago was subtitled 'Mining for silver while dreaming of gold' (2001). That metaphor was used to convey the proposition that although CDM studies are not 'gold standard' randomised controlled experiments, they could still make significant contributions to knowledge for the field, for the organisation in which they are conducted and for the practitioner researchers who conduct them. In my admittedly biased opinion, this rich and varied collection of CDM studies by allied health practitioners amply supports the foregoing proposition. However, in the end, it is for the exceptional writers of this collection and its readers to make the final judgement.

Irwin Epstein, PhD
H Rehr Professor of Applied Social Work Research
(Health & Mental Health)
Hunter College School of Social Work
City University of New York

References

Epstein I (2010). *Clinical data-mining: integrating practice and research*. New York: Oxford University Press.

Epstein I (2001). Using available clinical information in practice-based research: mining for silver when dreaming of gold. In I Epstein & S Blumenfield (Eds). *Clinical data-mining in practice based research* (pp15–32). New York: The Haworth Social Work Press.

Epstein I & Blumenfield S (Eds) (2001). *Clinical data-mining in practice-based research*. New York: The Haworth Social Work Press.

Joubert L & Epstein I (Eds) (2005). Multi-disciplinary data-mining in allied health practice: another perspective on Australian research and evaluation. *Journal of Social Work Research and Evaluation* 6(2): 139–229.

Plath D & Gibbons J (2010). Discoveries on a data-mining expedition: single sessions social work in hospitals. *Social Work in Health Care* 49(8): 703–17.

Contributors

Chris Barnett is the senior physiotherapist, outpatient physiotherapy services at the Royal Newcastle Centre.

Phoebe Begg BSocSt (University of Sydney) is a social worker with Upper Hunter Community Health, based at Scone Health Services. This position provides generalist social work services to hospital inpatients and community clients. Phoebe's clinical interests are rural mental health, strength-based practice and practice-based research.

Sarah Bone BSpPath is a speech pathologist and research assistant at John Hunter Hospital which is part of Hunter New England Health. Clinical interests include voice disorders, irritable larynx syndrome and thyroid disease.

Lisa Channon BHSc (OccTherapy) (Hons) is the team leader for the Occupational Therapy Department at the John Hunter Hospital, within Hunter New England Health. Clinical interests include acute adult trauma presentations and the management of associated orthopaedic and traumatic brain injuries.

Carla Dyson was an honours physiotherapy student at the University of Newcastle. She currently works on the Gold Coast and collated and analysed the Allied Health Management Information System data as part of her honours dissertation.

Robert Eisenberg is the Director of the Department of Otolaryngology, Head and Neck Surgery, in Hunter New England Health and has a special interest in thyroid and parathyroid surgery.

Irwin Epstein MSW, PhD occupies the Helen Rehr Chair in Applied Social Work Research in Health and Mental Health at Hunter College School of Social Work of the City University of New York. In an international career devoted to collaboration between research academics and practitioners, he has co-authored several books and numerous articles on professionalisation, program evaluation, research utilisation and clinical data mining (CDM). Having introduced this latter concept and methodology into the social work and allied health professions, he continues to explore CDM as a strategy for engaging health and mental health practitioners in knowledge-building and as an alternative PhD research paradigm. His latest book on the subject is entitled *Clinical data-mining: integrating practice and research*, published in 2010 by Oxford University Press.

Roslyn Giles BSW (NSW), MSW (University of Newcastle), AM is currently a senior lecturer and the Director of Social Work Field Education at the University of Sydney. This role has bought together her extensive experiences as a social work practitioner and manager, as a field education supervisor and as a tertiary social work educator. Roslyn is very interested in how adult learners continuously combine their life experiences with formal processes of critical reflection and skill development, in striving to develop just and ethical human service practice. Her research includes projects to develop and implement national social work practice standards, as well as health context practice-based data-mining projects and research about social work priorities in practice.

Robin Haskins is a senior physiotherapist at the Royal Newcastle Centre, John Hunter Hospital.

Judith Henderson BAppSc (App. Phty), MAppSc (Manip. Phty) is the Area Profession Director, Physiotherapy, for Hunter New England Health; Director of Physiotherapy for Greater Newcastle Acute Hospital Network; Acting Service Manager Allied Health, Greater Newcastle Acute Hospital Network 2008 to present; and conjoint senior lecturer at the University of Newcastle. She also chairs the NSW Department of Health Physiotherapy Advisors Network.

Fran Hodgson BSW, MAppMgt (Health) is the Director of Social Work for the Greater Newcastle Acute Hospital Network and has been based at John Hunter Hospital for the past seven of her 26 years working in health. Fran gained extensive social work experience working with younger people with disabilities, aged care and dementia support and education before moving into health management roles for the last 10 years. She has been involved in social work outcomes projects since 2005.

Gabrielle Murphy BSW is a social worker with extensive experience in the field of hepatitis C treatment and management, having worked in the John Hunter Hospital Hepatology Service for nine years. She is currently working at the Hunter Institute of Mental Health, developing a core skills training package for mental health clinicians in Hunter New England Mental Health. Clinical interests include short and long-term social and mental health implications of hepatitis C and its treatment, as well as in social work and allied health outcomes.

Peter Osmotherly has over 20 years of clinical experience as a physiotherapist. He is also qualified in clinical epidemiology and has completed research using various methodologies. He is currently a senior lecturer at the University of Newcastle.

Luisa Renna BSpPath is a Level 3 speech pathologist working with acute adult caseloads and specialising in acute stroke rehabilitation. Particular interests include swallowing and communication management with acute stroke and progressive neurological populations.

David Rhodes was the Area Director of Allied Health in the then Hunter New England Area Health Service for a 10-year period. His position allowed for the strategic development of an allied health profile within the area and at state and national levels. His position created professional supports across the area, including the establishment of professional leadership roles in each profession, the attraction of funding for recurrent service enhancements and operational infrastructure, and promoting allied health research activities. David was also the inaugural Director of Health Professionals at the Canberra Hospital, ACT, for a 10-year period and has worked extensively in community health and rehabilitation services. David contributed to the development of the National Allied Health Benchmarking Consortium, the National Allied Health Classification Committee and Allied Health Professions Australia. He is currently the Assistant Director, Allied Health, Nursing and Midwifery, in the NSW Health Professional Councils Authority.

Kate Rutledge BAppSc (App. Phty) is a senior physiotherapist in the Greater Newcastle Acute Hospital Network (GNAHN).

Christine Smith BAppSc (App. Phty) is acting team leader physiotherapist in the Greater Newcastle Acute Hospital Network (GNAHN).

Damien Smith BAppSc (App. Phty), Bach. of Nurs. is acting team leader physiotherapist, Greater Newcastle Acute Hospital Network (GNAHN).

Jenny Swancott BSocSt (University of Sydney), Master of Social Work (University of Newcastle) is a senior social worker and team leader at the Royal Newcastle Centre, Greater Newcastle Acute Hospital Network. Jenny was initially employed as a school social worker. Her hospital experience includes seven years in oncology, with the last 17 years in orthopaedic rehabilitation, encompassing musculoskeletal injuries, spinal cord injuries and chronic pain.

Sarah Thompson Dip OT is an occupational therapist in the Upper Hunter, Hunter New England Health. She is also an executive councillor of the NSW Farmers Association, Chair of Rural Affairs Committee, participating in the NSW Farmers Mental Health Network. Interests include paediatric developmental issues, rural health and overcoming farm clients' isolation from pathways to health, particularly in the area of mental health and impacts of drought.

Anne Vertigan BAppSc (Sp Path), MBA, PhD is the area profession director for speech pathology for Hunter New England Local Clinical Network, director for speech pathology with the Greater Newcastle Acute Hospital Network and conjoint lecturer at the University of Newcastle. She is also chair of the Hunter New England Health Allied Health Research Committee. Clinical interests include voice disorders, dysphagia and irritable larynx syndrome.

Glade Vyslysel BA, MA (Occupational Therapy) is an occupational therapist/team leader working for Hunter New England Health. Clinical interests include working with adults with acquired brain injury. Glade has a strong interest in bridging the practice–evidence gap by contributing to research projects while maintaining a role as a full-time practising clinician.

Introduction

Roslyn Giles, Anne E Vertigan, Irwin Epstein and David Rhodes

This book presents the results of an eight-year practice-based research (PBR) capacity building project aiming to support allied health practitioners in their efforts to take up current health challenges of evidence-based practice (EBP) and the demonstration of healthcare needs, practices and outcomes. The book demonstrates many of the achievements of this unique capacity building project undertaken by multiple allied health practitioners working in single disciplinary and multidisciplinary teams in an Australian allied health setting.

The choice of a clinical data-mining (CDM) approach was inspired by the series of International Social Work in Health and Mental Health conferences presenting CDM research projects by practitioners and academics from the US, Israel and Australia. The combination of a rigorous research methodology, practice-based evidence, a realistic practice focus and achievable practitioner-research processes encouraged Hunter New England Allied Health leaders to adopt a similar approach.

The health service environment

Today's health service environment is one of increasing demands for service provision accompanied by shrinking budgets and consistent organisational restructure. In this environment, health professionals face increasing demands for accountability in relation to the effectiveness and outcomes of interventions (Gray & Muir 1997). This contemporary emphasis on EBP requires all practitioners to focus on the arenas where their knowledge and skills achieve the most effective outcomes and the best value for expenditure.

In providing effective and person-centred services the reflective practitioner (Argyris & Schon 1976) of the past is now becoming the reflective practitioner researcher. The reflective practitioner researcher is a professional, whose job description encompasses both service provision and research, creating the questions for research from their experiences of practice. Central to this evolution is a breaking down of the longstanding dichotomy separating research and practice. Research, traditionally confined to the context of academia and the skills of a highly qualified researcher, is evolving into strong practice and academic partnerships. In these partnerships it is the practitioner who plays a lead role in creating and researching practice-relevant questions rather than research questions being generated from the detached theorist (Fook 2002). In this era of the practitioner researcher, research is now viewed as a core professional skill (D'Cruz & Jones 2004). While critical reflection, practice wisdom and expert processes of decision-making about appropriate professional actions remain essential to wise and effective practice (Plath 2006), this wisdom now needs to be clearly based in research which objectively demonstrates the basis of decisions in relation to both direct individual client interventions as well as the programs and services provided. In such a research-focused practice environment, allied health professionals have worked to increase practitioner research capacity. The creation of education opportunities and networks of support has encouraged allied health practitioners in their evolution into integrated practitioner researchers. This book demonstrates the outcome of one such organisational research learning process.

Allied health

The concept of allied health is well developed in Australia. Allied health professions are known as those clinical healthcare professions distinct from medicine, nursing and dentistry. Working alongside and independently of medicine, nursing and dentistry, allied health professions are core to the provision of holistic health services. In Australia these 90,000-plus allied health professionals include the following disciplines: audiologists, chiropractors, dietitians, exercise physiologists, occupational therapists, orthoptists, orthotists and prosthetists, osteopaths, pharmacists, podiatrists, physiotherapists, psychologists, radiographers, radiation therapists and sonographers, social workers, speech pathologists and a number of small professions such as music therapists and genetic counsellors (Allied Health Professionals Australia AHPA 2007). Allied health professionals require a tertiary degree which includes supervised clinical placements. In recent years there has been more organisational recognition of allied health in state and territory government structures through the appointment of Chief Allied Health Officers, the creation of Director of Allied Health management positions in public sector organisations, the formation of national allied health organisations such as Allied Health Professions Australia (AHPA) and Services for Australian Rural and Remote Allied Health (SARRAH) and specific recommendations on allied health from government investigations and commissions of inquiry. Additionally, allied health professions have been recognised in improved industrial awards including the NSW Health Service Health Professionals (State) Award.

The concept of 'allied health' has been well documented in the literature over the past two decades as evidenced by the writings of Boyce (1993, 2001, 2004, 2006), Turnbull et al. (2009) and Law and Boyce (2003) among others.

The practitioner researcher

Fundamentally no different to any other researcher, the practitioner researcher aims to ask questions and generate new knowledge. However, as a curious and questioning professional, the practitioner researcher seeks rigorous and objective methods to answer questions generated directly from their work with the people they aim to serve and from their service setting. Whilst having similar aims to academic researchers, the practitioner researcher is in a unique position in the research process. They have direct access to the child or adult, have daily experiences with these people's concerns and needs, and keep data recording and evaluating these experiences. The practitioner researcher is the professional who moves from introspection and dialogue about the details of their practice, its complexities and process, from the wellbeing of their clients and associated problem solving, to objective, systematic research data collection and analysis.

In this position, the practitioner researcher can embed research in a manner that an academic researcher cannot. Often viewing themselves as less important than an academic researcher, practitioner researchers can minimise their vital role in the development of new knowledge and the testing of academic research in the real and unique world of people and services. On the contrary, the place and nature of the practitioner researcher is now essential in seeking to understand and improve the work of public health allied health practitioners. Genuine theory and knowledge can only be generated through practice in the reality of the people and circumstances to whom the knowledge is relevant (Jarvis 1999; Fox et al. 2007).

Building research capacity

In facing the challenges of becoming reflective practitioner researchers, professionals are encouraged to consider underpinning influences supporting the processes of learning in practice. Immersing themselves in the business of daily practice of providing client-focused services, it is also essential to reflect on how the organisational structure, culture and approach to learning and new knowledge can simultaneously support, challenge and change the reflective practitioner researcher. In the process of this capacity-building research project, discussions of influential dynamics have provided valuable reflections about why the integration of research into this daily practice has at times seemed an insurmountable struggle.

Organisational culture

Consideration of organisational culture invites contemplation of the dominant nature and characteristics of an organisation in the same manner as we might reflect on the nature and characteristics of ethnic groups and nations. Handy (1993) invites consideration of how power, roles, tasks and personal natures influence actions and outcomes in organisations. The communication of these elements influences the spoken and unspoken messages about 'the way things are done around here'. Such communication can promote a culture of learning and excellence or it can reduce some practitioners to being handmaidens not expected to take a prominent place in reflection, thinking and new ways of practising.

Organisational learning

Central to an encouraging and empowering organisational culture is the concept of organisational learning. Senge (2000) notes that the process of learning, developing and changing within large and complex organisations can at times be fraught with difficulties.

> The way organisations are designed and managed, the way people's jobs are defined, the way we are taught to think and interact (not only in organisations but more broadly) create fundamental disabilities. These disabilities operate despite the best efforts of committed people. (Senge 2000, p.18)

Counterbalancing such depleting experiences of organisational dynamics is understanding how organisations are also able to be reflective, learn and change. Giddens (1984) encourages practitioners to be informed about the processes of power and influence between practitioners and their organisational base. An analysis of the combined factors of repeated human actions leads practitioners to recognise that if humans change their actions it is possible to transform organisational structures, a process Giddens refers to as structuration.

Senge (2000) takes Giddens' notion of 'structuration' into real actions, claiming that learning organisations are active in creating, capturing, transferring and mobilising knowledge to enable it to adapt to a changing environment. Learning organisations do not rely on passive or unconsidered processes in the hope that change will occur. Rather, learning organisations strongly promote, facilitate and reward collective learning, contributing to valued and essential change. In changing their action Senge (2000) encourages practitioners to address four core principles of learning organisations – personal mastery, mental models, shared vision and team learning.

Transformational learning

Creating organisational cultures with shared visions for research in practice and team learning opportunities that assist practitioners to work differently within powerful structures is important for team development. However, critically reflective practitioners will also move beyond external assumptions and meanings of organisational learning and change their personal, internal processes for learning and changing their practice. While the individual nature of learning style is well recognised, Jarvis' (2006) adult learning research demonstrates that essential to the process of practitioner growth and development are opportunities for new practice experiences combined with internal and social reflection. If this new learning is to be more than transitory (i.e. to have a deep and lasting impact that changes practice actions to enhance the wellbeing of patients and clients), practitioner researchers require significant learning experiences that engage them intellectually, emotionally and socially. Defined as transformational learning, this process moves the practitioner researcher learner beyond the attainment of factual knowledge into his/her own experience, thinking and meaning making. The practitioner researcher has opportunities to reflect on and analyse their learning, build onto their previous learning, and assess the relevance of this learning for a future situation (Giles et al. 2010). In so doing, learning practitioner researchers develop a sense of personal mastery, a personal confidence in the skills and knowledge of practice research. Accompanied by mental models about how to undertake research in practice and team support for reflection and new knowledge creation, the critically reflective practitioner becomes the critically reflective practitioner researcher.

Why clinical data mining?

Simply stated, CDM is a form of practice-based research (PBR) in which practitioners locate, extract, analyse and interpret available clinical data for practice knowledge-building, clinical decision-making and reflective practice (Epstein 2001). CDM is an evidence-based approach whereby practitioners can reflect on their own practice by systematically researching existing information.

What sets CDM apart from conventional evidence-based practice (EBP) is that EBP treats practitioners as mere consumers and appliers of research knowledge generated by researchers other than themselves (Epstein 2009; Epstein & Joubert 2010). By contrast, CDM empowers practitioners as co-contributors to knowledge about their own practice using their own practice-based evidence (Epstein 2010).

In allied health practice, practitioners routinely collect and record enormous quantities of information about patient characteristics, worker interventions and patient responses to these interventions. These records provide potentially rich sources of data for research, data that are rarely 'mined' by either researchers or practitioners.

Although CDM relies on 'gold-standard' experimental logic, it requires neither randomisation nor control groups. It makes use of both qualitative and quantitative data and data-analytic techniques, and does not intrude on service delivery. Perhaps most importantly, it welcomes practice wisdom as a basis for knowledge development and testing. Practical wisdom in professional practice requires sound judgment in the use of personal/professional, theoretical and practical knowledge (Goodfellow 2002). Wisdom has been described as a way of knowing, involving expert knowledge and sound judgment along with having reflective and moral/ethical qualities. Practical wisdom combines personal qualities, practical knowledge, sound judgment and thoughtful action (Goodfellow 2002). The independent living unit (ILU) chapter demonstrates many years of practice wisdom where practitioner actions were recognised as contributing to good patient outcomes. However, a deeper level of analysis of these practitioner actions has revealed further valuable knowledge for improved practice.

Data mining is commonly used in very sophisticated ways in the business sector where many industries recognise that existing records are a rich data source to support decision-making. The concept of CDM and CDM methods were introduced and developed over a decade ago by Epstein (2001, 2007) at the Mount Sinai Medical Centre in New York. Since then, CDM has been successfully employed by individual practitioners, social work units and multidisciplinary teams in health, mental health and child welfare services in multiple settings and several countries (Joubert & Epstein 2005; Epstein & Joubert 2010). Additionally, CDM has been used in PhD research projects by practitioners seeking academic careers (Epstein 2010). Each of these studies has led to significant discoveries and made valuable contributions to understanding practice within and beyond the agency in which it was conducted. Many have become the bases for professional conference presentations and peer-reviewed publications by the practitioners who conducted them. All have enhanced practitioner reflection, research skills and professional self-esteem.

Perhaps more important than publications or conference presentations, CDM encourages practitioners to be more reflective about their practice and to use practice-based evidence and research in their practice decision-making. CDM practitioner researchers begin every project by asking questions about what they do, why they do it, how outcomes might be measured, and how well they are achieving these outcomes. Next, CDM provides achievable methodologies for identifying existing qualitative and quantitative data sources, data extraction and analyses with the ultimate aim of providing better and more efficient services to patients.

In providing an achievable applied research ideology and methodology, CDM enables the performance of a number of functions. These include providing a query for clinical conditions, extracting related information, and knowledge discovery. Accordingly, the purposes of CDM can be summarised as to:

- refine and enhance practice wisdom
- describe and evaluate practice
- promote evidence-informed practice
- identify best practices
- promote evidence-informed reflective practice by the practitioner
- promote team-building and pride in professionalism.

Advantages of CDM

Many academic researchers reflexively reject the use of existing clinical data for research purposes and there may be sound methodological reasons for their caution. Their reasons usually involve the quality and incompleteness of the data available and problems of reliability and validity (Kagle 1996; Reamer 1998). However, existing records may be more valuable and potentially useful than initially thought. In some disciplines, for example, standardised measures are used routinely in clinical assessment and outcome evaluation. In others, there are limited standardised measures or they are too cumbersome to use. In some of these practice contexts, existing data is better than nothing or intrusively collecting original standardised data (Chan et al. 2009). EBP advocates express further concerns about the scientific rigour with which practitioners make judgements about patients (Pignotti & Thyer 2009). Although bias must be considered and accounted for, one must not discount the fact that clinicians are trained, qualified and paid to make such clinical judgements in day-to-day practice. And it is these judgements that significantly affect the fates of their patients.

CDM encourages practitioners to reflect on the basis of their own decisions and the outcomes associated with those decisions. While undertaking rigorous reflection and research, CDM does not require clinicians to do anything with patients that they do not already do. It is not intrusive and patients do not interact with any research agenda. CDM enlists practitioners in obtaining data samples and maintaining the integrity of the study design. While being practitioner-driven CDM may require methodological consultation. Even then, it is the practitioner rather than the research consultant who determines the interesting questions of their data. Practitioners remain active at every step in the CDM process; they are not simply used to do the drudge work of research or the enlistment of research subjects. Such studies can lead to evidence-based changes in the way services are delivered (Epstein & Blumenfield 2001).

As a legitimate research methodology CDM can be conceptualised as evidence-informed practice (Epstein 2009). Although academic research critics find this objectionable (Auslander 2010), CDM does not commence with a literature review. It begins with practice wisdom about practice-based problems, practice reflection and clinicians' inductive and conceptual exploration of the problem. It is methodologically pluralist and is compatible with both qualitative and quantitative data. The literature review is conducted later to confirm, refute or explain their findings. This is one of several ways in which CDM involves a 'strategic compromise' between research ideals and practice realities (Epstein 2010). In so doing CDM offers the advantage of being possible where the ideal is not achievable (Epstein 2001), and for the inquiring practitioner CDM provides a research process that brings together the tensions of critical reflection and evidence-based practice (Plath 2006).

For beginning practice researchers, CDM can be used to simply describe and evaluate practice. It is extremely important for practitioners to know what other practitioners are doing. How faithfully are programs being followed? Is the model of care being adhered to? What is the patient group being served and what needs do they bring? Is there a difference in background characteristics, problems presented, services received and health outcomes? These are questions that every practitioner should be asking and answering with their own data.

In moving from practice wisdom to research, CDM also helps practitioners articulate and empirically test practice-based knowledge. Without rigorous review and analysis, practitioners may be misguided in their unsystematic observations. Practitioner perceptions and actions can focus on the atypical and challenging patient problems skewing their overall perspectives. In CDM, 'outlier' cases are not ignored but are collated into the total picture of a patient population. This will be seen in the chapter on thyroid services where services to a subgroup were nearly disbanded based on inaccurate practitioner impressions whereas the data showed that a significant proportion of patients required further services.

More generally, CDM is useful to practitioners who are interested in learning about their own practice. For example, a speech pathologist working with patients who have dysphagia (swallowing disorders) may be interested in patterns of clinical features associated with patients requiring texture modified diets. CDM is an evidence-based approach for answering these questions.

In contrast with business uses of data mining which are very sophisticated, statistical methods routinely employed by practitioners in CDM are relatively simple. Extracted data can be recorded onto readily available spreadsheet programs and exported into statistical packages for analysis. Practitioners are encouraged to start with simple statistics such as percentages, t-tests, chi squares and other conventional measures of association. Nonetheless, in doctoral dissertations the more sophisticated statistical procedures and research designs used in business applications have been shown to be applicable (Epstein 2010).

Clinicians interested in commencing quality assurance (QA) or practice-based research projects may be encouraged to begin by identifying what data they already have rather than assuming that they must collect original data to answer their questions. The chapter on farming families commenced with a simple quality review question and database and later progressed into a full research project. This project is also an example of CDM as both a retrospective and prospective methodology (Epstein & Joubert 2010). It also demonstrates how extracting data from one's own records encourages practitioners to become better future record-keepers.

Ultimately CDM rests on the basic assumption that practitioners are interested in learning from their mistakes as well as their successes. In so doing, it puts into practice the concept of a learning organisation (Epstein 2010) and CDM aids practitioners with the sometimes blurry lines between research and QA by providing a direct link between QA and PBR.

Pitfalls of CDM

As with any other research strategy, there are a number of pitfalls associated with CDM that warrant consideration. Firstly, the retrospective nature of CDM means that desired data may not be available. CDM practitioners are reliant on the scope and quality of previously collected data. In other words, there may be missing data; for example, gender or weight not routinely collected in all patients in the sample, or data was never designed to be collected, such as race or height. Secondly, CDM can be labour intensive and requires commitment of time and energy.

CDM may be criticised by experimentalists as not sufficiently rigorous. Likewise, some EBP advocates assert that reliance on 'usual practice' is inherently dangerous or even undesirable if not demonstrated through a randomised trial (Gambrill 2010). However, there are many situations where a randomised trial is undesirable or impractical. Mouth-to-mouth resuscitation after drowning is a prime example of where randomising to a 'no-treatment' group would be unthinkable. In most instances, it is essential to understand the current practice and its outcomes in order to formulate targeted improvement activities and consequent research on changed practice and its impact.

The complementary relationships between PBR, CDM and EBP

Table 1 demonstrates the complementary relationship between PBR, CDM and EBP while placing CDM in the context of EBP. Concerns have been expressed about potential misinterpretations of EBP and the messages that go to practitioners from promoters of EBP. EBP provides practitioners with the evidence that others have gathered, analysed and published and is intended to contribute to a *universal* body of knowledge. However, it is important not to obscure or dilute *local* knowledge that is more directly applicable to the cultural and organisational context in which specific sets of practitioners work (Epstein et al. 2010). Moreover, by disparaging practice wisdom and discounting less than 'gold standard' practitioner research, EBP can create an artificial and unfortunate division of labour between clinicians and researchers. Clinicians have a greater role and contribution than simply implementing clinical practice guidelines developed by researchers. Reflective and considered clinicians have a pivotal role in the acquisition of knowledge (Plath 2006; Epstein 2009).

Research findings must be contextualised to the patient group and setting. Evidence-based practice is about universal guidelines in terms of what suits the majority of patients with a particular condition. It invokes the valuable concept of best practice. However, the outliers are common, particularly in public health systems. Although these outliers might provide important information about a condition or treatment, they are often ignored or even excluded from EBP analysis. Given that outliers can consume considerable resources in the health setting, they may warrant more intense investigation. CDM provides one means to examine the outlier impact on clinical and health systems experience. The chapter on the hepatitis C trifecta demonstrates the vital nature of local new knowledge when global research results are considered at the local public health level.

CDM is not in competition with EBP. It is on a continuum with other research methodologies, each with its own strengths and limitations. Rather, CDM is an alternative approach that has utility in specific situations. Before EBP had reached its current popularity, Epstein distinguished between research-based models of practice knowledge development and practice-based models (PBR) (Epstein 2001). EBP may be considered a particular form of research-based practice (RBP). There are a number of distinct differences between RBP or evidence-based practice and practice-based research (PBR). Firstly, RBP is deductive and theory driven whereas PBR is inductive and relies on practice wisdom of the researcher. Secondly, RBP seeks to confirm or refute causation particularly through use of randomised control trials (RCT). The aim is to prove or disprove that treatment is effective and is important for removing bias. In contrast, PBR describes correlation and may not be the best design to answer questions of causation. A third difference between RBP and PBR refers to the type of data analysis. RBP is predominantly quantitative whereas PBR can use a combination of quantitative and qualitative data.

In fact the following chapters in this book attest to the range of data types that can be collected using CDM methodology, ranging from clinician and patient experiences of treatment to specific instrumental measures used in voice testing. RBP is summative whereas PBR is formative. RBP is research driven and *may* be collaborative between researcher and clinician. In contrast PBR tends to be more fully collaborative, practice driven and often inspired by the experiences and questions of the clinicians. In fact it can be the frustrations experienced by clinicians with unanswered questions in the literature that can inspire PBR initiatives (Epstein 2009).

Ultimately each research paradigm is essential to best practice, with the large-scale control group methodologies providing best practice guidelines and the practitioner-based research addressing the unique experiences of local applications while stimulating the development of new knowledge (see Table 1). Rather than viewing CDM among the lower ranks in the evidence hierarchy where RCT is considered at the peak followed by quasi experimental studies, correlation studies, qualitative studies and case studies, it could be considered alongside these methodologies as a valid approach in particular situations. These various research methodologies could be considered as part of a wheel of evidence incorporating each of the methodologies.

Hunter New England Health: the organisational context

In Hunter New England Health (HNE) in New South Wales, Australia, clinical services are available for approximately 840,000 people. It covers a geographical area of over 130,000 square kilometres equivalent to the landmass of England. It has approximately 14,500 staff including 1500 medical officers, 1100 allied health and has 1600 volunteers. HNE provides services to 12% of the state's population and to 20% of the state's Aboriginal population. It spans 25 local council areas. HNE is unique, in that it is the only health district in NSW with a major metropolitan centre (Newcastle/Lake Macquarie) as well as a mix of several large regional centres and many smaller rural centres and remote communities within its borders. Allied health staff work in most clinical settings – hospitals, community health centres, rehabilitation centres, home-based services and population-based programs.

The Area Director of Allied Health role was created in 2000. Prior to the creation of this position there was no-one to lead allied health strategically in areas such as strategic planning, service review and design, research, statistics and information management, continuity of care, and innovative service models. Limited data were collected using standardised data elements, and most departments and professions had no electronic data collection and care management systems. In 2001, the Allied Health Management Information System (AHMIS)

Table 1. Comparison of evidence-based practice, practice-based research (PBR) and clinical data mining

Research paradigm	General application	Strengths	Limitations
Evidence-based practice	Provides practitioners with evidence that others have gathered, analysed and published	Contributes to a universal body of knowledge	Obscures and dilutes local knowledge
	Provides universal guidelines in terms of what suits the majority of patients with a particular condition	Analyses causation on a large scale	Creates an artificial division of labour between clinicians and researchers
	Predominantly quantitative methodologies	Provides sound information about treatment efficacy	Ignores outliers and the unique
		Utilises randomisation which ensures participant characteristics are consistent across groups.	May not report on the findings of subsets
		Reduces allocation bias	
		Allows blinding	

Research paradigm	General application	Strengths	Limitations
Practitioner-based research	Inductive and relies on practice wisdom of the researcher	Fully collaborative, practice driven and often inspired by the experiences and questions of the clinicians	May not be the best design to answer questions of causation
	Combines qualitative and quantitative methodologies		
Clinical data mining	A form of PBR in which practitioners locate, extract, analyse and interpret available clinical data for practice knowledge-building, clinical decision-making and reflective practice	An evidence-based approach where practitioners can reflect on their own practice by systematically researching the information they already have	Desired data may not always be available
		Provides a rigorous methodology for researching local practices	Labour intensive and requires commitment of time and energy
		Can report on the findings of subsets	Criticised by experimentalists as not sufficiently rigorous
			Does not answer questions of causality

was implemented which was the first standardised data collection system in acute settings in HNE. Subsequently the Community Health Information Management Enterprise (CHIME), a care management system, was introduced that aids in the collation of community-based allied health data as a byproduct of routine clinical practice. Both these systems established the ground for well considered and rigorous allied health practice-based research (PBR) across the continuum of care.

CDM infrastructure

Health-based clinical research in allied health has progressed over the last decade. Allied health staff participate in projects either as project leaders and coordinators, multidisciplinary team members, or assist with data collection (Joubert & Epstein 2005). There are relatively few clinical research positions in allied health in Australia and therefore most staff undertaking research projects must juggle existing clinical and administrative roles. There are a number of challenges to allied health staff in completing research projects, including competing clinical demands, lack of funding, lack of skills in research methodology and an absence of dedicated research time.

The HNE Allied Health Research Committee was established in 2002. The committee comprised the Area Director of Allied Health and a representative from each of the allied health disciplines of nutrition and dietetics, occupational therapy, podiatry, speech pathology, social work, psychology and physiotherapy. Meetings were held once a month. The purpose of the committee was to facilitate allied health and multidisciplinary research, increase the research skill base of allied health staff and to develop an infrastructure to support research for allied health staff, including projects done in conjunction with multidisciplinary teams. The responsibility and scope of activities of the committee was to:

a. seek out funding opportunities for projects including availability of grants

b. assist staff with preparation of submissions and ethics proposals

c. promote research activities of allied health staff

d. develop a network of resources to support allied health in research

e. make recommendations regarding distribution of research funding

f. develop a long-term strategy for education, liaison and process

g. formalise links with the local university through development of a memorandum of association

h. facilitate education for staff regarding research through an active learning model

i. formalise processes for research amongst allied health staff and catalogue activities and outputs

j. apply for research grants and assist other staff to prepare research grants

k. assist staff in research design

l. monitor progress of research initiatives in the area and provide support and assistance

m. facilitate education on research methodology

n. provide recommendations regarding allocation of funding

o. organise an annual research forum and clinical data-mining workshops

p. encourage staff to develop projects of a multidisciplinary nature

q. facilitate research mentoring.

At the time of commencement of the committee, allied health research was infrequent and allied health staff faced a number of barriers to conducting research. These barriers included difficulties juggling competing roles, insufficient clinical backfill to complete research, insufficient training in research skills and insufficient statistical knowledge. The research committee did not have a formal budget but was able to fund a small number of projects.

The committee encouraged each profession to develop a methodology and to draft a proposal for a potential project in the event that grants or funding became available at short notice. The committee organised annual research forums to provide education about research methodology and an opportunity to showcase research that has been conducted. Finally, a register was developed to record completed research projects, and projects in various stages of development. The register was published on the HNE intranet to enhance collaboration, mentoring and engagement in the research agenda. The committee provides individual and group consultation sessions with researchers and has coordinated clinical data-mining activities in the region since 2005. Surveys of allied health staff conducted in 2003 and 2009 found that there has been improved backfill for research, greater involvement in research and improved training in clinical skills.

CDM in Australian allied health

The concept of CDM was initially launched in the Hunter region at a multidisciplinary workshop in Newcastle, Australia, in 2005 with Professor Irwin Epstein of Hunter College New York and Dr Lynette Joubert of the University of Melbourne. The session was attended by over 100 staff from health, academia and community services. Following this launch, clinical data-mining workshops have been conducted on an annual basis. The workshops were funded by the Area Director of Allied Health for HNE.

In preparation for the workshops, individuals or teams submitted CDM project proposals to the Allied Health Research Committee. These proposals ranged from ideas of potential projects, to projects in progress and projects using existing complete datasets. The research committee then scheduled consultation sessions for the projects between Professor Epstein and each individual or team. The structure of the consultation session involved a brief presentation from the team followed by a 10–15 minute question and advice session.

In addition to the formal consultation sessions, a lecture was given during each workshop on the background and methodology of CDM. These lectures were attended by a range of allied health professionals, medical and administration staff. The lectures were also available to clinicians in rural areas via videoconferencing. Following each of Epstein's education and consultation sessions, Anne Vertigan (HNE) and Roslyn Giles (Social Work, University of Sydney) provided mentoring and support to the practice researchers.

Results: what was achieved

A number of CDM projects have been undertaken; many of them are reported in the following chapters of this book. There was a range of professions presenting projects. A summary of projects presented during consultation sessions is shown in Table 2.

Although many projects were concluded and reported, a number of projects did not continue through to completion. Reasons for non-completion included changing in staffing and positions; failing to find clinically significant findings that would be of interest beyond the setting; or that, once commenced, the research area was no longer a clinical or organisational priority.

A number of professional findings have been determined following commencement of these projects, and many are reported in subsequent chapters. The findings have influenced decisions about clinical prioritisation and service provision. Other examples of such projects have already been published (Wickham et al. 2010). Plath and Gibbons employed CDM with hospital social workers to explore the use and outcomes of short single-session contacts with clients in an acute hospital context. This work demonstrates the value and limitations of brief contacts under pressure. The Nutrition and Dietetics department initially employed clinical data-mining methodology to investigate malnutrition in hospital inpatients. This project eventually extended beyond CDM methodology and informed the new EQuIP5 Criterion 1.5.7 (safety standard), influencing the New South Wales Health Nutrition Standards for adult inpatients. The project has also enabled the Nutrition Care Policy and participation in the Australia-wide AuSPEN Nutrition Care Day Survey. The department has also received an innovations scholarship for the 'Eating matters: protected mealtimes' project. These outcomes have all stemmed from the work begun in 2005 (Watterson et al. 2009). In addition to profession- and team-specific knowledge development, there has been an increase in the collective skill base of allied health staff and the Allied Health Research Committee. These skills have enhanced the capacity of the research teams

Table 2. Projects presented during consultation sessions

Profession	Project	Year
Nutrition and dietetics	Malnutrition	2006
	Nutritional management in hospitalised stroke patients	2008
	PEG tube complications	2008
Speech pathology	Carer communication groups	2006
	Multidisciplinary tracheostomy care	2006 & 2007
	Scoping current practice in chronic cough management	2006
	Inpatient assessment tool for swallowing	2006
	Thyroid surgery	2007
	Aphasia assessment results in acute care	2008
Social work	Farming families	2006, 2007 & 2008
	Social isolation in the elderly	2006
	Living with arthritis	2007
	Independent living unit	2007
	Social work outcomes project	2007
	Hepatitis C psychosocial assessment database	2008
	Supporting parents after removal of baby	2008
Physiotherapy	Testing AHMIS/CHIME codeset for outpatient services	2006
	Low back pain	2007
Podiatry	Hypergranulation tissue	2007

to provide straightforward consultations to allied health staff regarding CDM and to facilitate the uptake of this methodology within allied health teams. Indeed access to CDM methodology may be a critical factor in determining whether or not quality and research activities can progress.

Further to projects such as these, some groups have taken steps to develop a new or expanded database prior to undertaking CDM projects. This has resulted in the development of a social work outcomes tool, now being further worked into an allied health outcome tool. This tool collates client-driven data about goals and outcomes of individual practitioner's interventions. The collation of this data provides vital information about the effectiveness of interventions with specific client groups, both for the individual practitioners and multidisciplinary teams.

Workshops and ongoing dialogue about research methods and skills have spurred practitioners to address their quality review processes and contribute to organisational and wider practitioner/academic research and quality review forums and conferences. Many of the projects have been presented in annual allied research forums, at national and international conferences.

Ethics and CDM

The issue of ethics approval for research is important and the rights and wellbeing of research participants is paramount. This, however, can create logistical complexities for researchers and the process of obtaining ethical approval for research projects can be extensive. The Hunter New England Human Research Ethics Committee provides ethical review of research in the district health service. This committee has advised that there are no ethics requirements for in-house data-mining projects as it is considered an appropriate research methodology. The situation can become complex with shared data and for publication of projects. Using de-identified data may be a feasible option. Two members of the allied health research committee are on the research ethics committee and this enables good understanding of the requirements of research ethics. In practice, prospective researchers in HNE have been encouraged to contact the professional officer of the committee for advice on whether projects require formal ethical review.

Conclusion

In summary, CDM can be considered a plausible strategy for QA and PBR projects. It is not a replacement of other research methods but an appropriate and achievable research methodology for many practice questions. In the Hunter region, training and ongoing support in CDM has strengthened allied health research culture. It has encouraged practitioner and organisational learning, client-focused service improvement and professional role satisfaction.

References

Allied Health Professionals Australia (2007). 2007 annual report. [Online]. Available: www.ahpa.com.au/pdfs/Annual_Report_2007.pdf [Accessed 25 March 2011].

Argyris C & Schon D (1976). *Theory in practice: increasing professional effectiveness*. San Francisco: Jossey-Bass.

Auslander G (2010). Book review of Epstein I. (2010) *Clinical data-mining: integrating practice and research*. New York: Oxford University Press. In *Social Work in Health Care*, 49: 764–67.

Boyce RA (2006). Emerging from the shadow of medicine: allied health as a 'profession community' subculture. *Health Sociology Review*, 15(5): 520–34.

Boyce RA (2004). The allied health professions in transition. In M Clinton (Ed). *Management in the Australian health care industry* (pp164–87). 3rd edn. Frenchs Forest NSW: Pearson Education Australia (Prentice Hall).

Boyce RA (2001). Organisational governance structures in allied health services: a decade of change. *Australian Health Review*, 24(1): 22–36.

Boyce RA (1993). Internal market reforms of health care systems and the allied health professions: an international perspective. *International Journal of Health Planning and Management*, 8: 201–17.

Chan WCH, Epstein I, Reese D & Chan CLW (2009). Family predictors of psycho-social outcomes among Hong Kong Chinese cancer patients in palliative care: living and dying with the support paradox. *Social Work in Health Care*, 48(5): 519–32.

D'Cruz H & Jones M (2004). *Social work research: ethical and political contexts*. London: Sage.

Epstein I (2010). *Clinical data-mining: integrating practice and research*. New York: Oxford University Press.

Epstein I (2009). Promoting harmony where there is commonly conflict: evidence-informed practice as an integrative strategy. *Social Work in Health Care*, 48(3): 216–31.

Epstein I (2007). From evaluation methodologist to clinical data-miner: finding treasure through practice-based research. In H Rehr & G Rosenberg (Eds). *The social work – medicine relationship: 100 years at Mount Sinai* (pp107–11). Binghamton, New York: The Haworth Social Work Press.

Epstein I (2001). Using available clinical information in practice-based research: mining for silver when dreaming of gold. In I Epstein & S Blumenfield (Eds). *Clinical data-mining in practice based research* (pp15–32). Binghamton, New York: The Haworth Social Work Press.

Epstein I & Blumenfield S (Eds) (2001). *Clinical data-mining in practice based research*. Binghamton, New York: The Haworth Social Work Press.

Epstein I & Joubert L (2010). Clinical data-mining in the age of evidence-based practice: recent exemplars and future challenges. In A Syvajarvi & J Stenvall (Eds). *Data mining in public and private sectors: organizational and government applications* (pp316–36). Hershey, New York: Information Science Reference.

Fook J (2002). Theorising from frontline practice: towards an inclusive approach for social work research. *Qualitative Social Work*, 1(1): 79–95.

Fox M, Martin P & Green G (2007). *Doing practitioner research*. London: Sage.

Gambrill E (2010). *Social work practice: a critical thinker's guide*. Oxford: Oxford University Press.

Giddens A (1984). *The constitution of society: outline of the theory of structuration.* Cambridge: Polity Press.

Giles R, Irwin J, Lynch D & Waugh F (2010). *In the field: learning to practice.* Melbourne: Oxford University Press.

Goodfellow, J (2002). Practical wisdom: exploring the hidden dimensions of professional practice. Paper presented at the Australian Association for Research in Education conference, Brisbane, December 2002.

Gray J & Muir A (1997). *Evidence based health care.* Edinburgh: Churchill Livingston.

Handy C (1993). *Understanding organisations.* 4th edn. Harmondsworth: Penguin.

Jarvis P (1999). *The practitioner researcher: developing theory from practice.* San Francisco: John Wiley & Sons.

Jarvis P (2006). *Towards a comprehensive theory of human learning.* New York: Routledge.

Joubert L & Epstein I (Eds) (2005). Multi-disciplinary data-mining in allied health practice: another perspective on Australian research and evaluation. Special Issue: *Journal of Social Work Research and Evaluation,* 6(2): 139–229.

Kagle JD (1996). *Social work records.* 2nd edn. Prospect Heights, IL: Waveland Press.

Law D & Boyce RA (2003). Beyond organisational design: moving from structure to service enhancement. *Australian Health Review,* 26(1): 161–71.

Plath D (2006). Evidenced-based practice: current issues and future debates. *Australian Social Work,* 59(1): 56–72.

Pignotti M & Thyer BA (2009). The use of novel unsupported and empirically supported therapies by licensed clinical social workers. *Social Work Research,* 33(1): 5–17.

Plath D & Gibbons J (2010). Discoveries on a data-mining expedition: single session social work in hospitals. *Social Work in Health Care,* 49(8): 703–17.

Reamer F (1998) *Social work research and evaluation skills: a case-based, user-friendly approach.* New York: Columbia University Press.

Senge P (2000). *The fifth discipline: the art and practice of the learning organisation.* Milsons Point: Random House.

Turnbull C, Grimmer-Somers K, Saravana Kumar K, May E, Law D & Ashworth E (2009). Allied, scientific and complementary health professionals: a new model for Australian allied health. *Australian Health Review*, 33(1): 27–37.

Watterson C, Frazer A, Banks M, Isenring E, Miller M, Silvester C, Hoevenaars R, Bauer J, Vivanti A & Ferguson M (2009). Evidence based practice guidelines for the nutritional management of malnutrition in adult patients across the continuum of care. *Nutrition and Dietetics 2009*, 66(Suppl 3): S1–S34. [Online]. Available: www.clinicalguidelines.gov.au/browse.php?treePath=&pageType=2&fld glrID=1617& [Accessed 25 March 2011].

Wickham M (2009). Who's left holding the woman? Practice issues facing hospital social workers working with women who have infants removed at birth by NSW Department of Community Services. *Children Australia*, 34(4): 29–35.

Chapter 1

A data-mining medley for physiotherapists: cleaning up data codes, evaluating service and improving client outcomes

Authors and project team: Judith Henderson, Christine Smith, Damien Smith, Chris Barnett, Robin Haskins and Kate Rutledge

Despite recommendations for data systems to better manage allied health services in acute facilities (NAHCC 2002), those that exist are not well developed. This limits the validity, reliability and utility of the clinical statistics they generate.

Hunter New England Health (HNE) Physiotherapy aimed to develop a 'data suite' providing relevant and complete information for the multiple purposes of organisational reporting, administration, benchmarking, data mining and clinical practice evaluation. This chapter presents three programmatic efforts to develop and trial codesets for medical diagnosis, clinical priority-setting and assessing clinical outcomes.

Key words: physiotherapy, codesets, research

The HNE Physiotherapy workforce is part of a large organisation, operating in the constantly changing wider health context of New South Wales (NSW), and Australia, and more broadly within international health and professional perspectives. Physiotherapy operates in HNE as a core allied health professional function involving approximately 370 practitioners across approximately 51 sites in the network.

Physiotherapy practice standards

Physiotherapists are responsible for demonstrating practice to acceptable standards (Australian Physiotherapy Council 2006). To demonstrate that their practice is faithful to acceptable standards, physiotherapists and physiotherapy services engage in ongoing improvement initiatives for clients and the wider health community. To achieve this, clinicians require tools to evaluate the 'fidelity' of their practice and to assist implementation of quality improvement practices.

One of the necessary tools for doing this is clean, accurate and relevant data, vital in terms of organisational, regional, state and national reporting of physiotherapy activities. These activities include quality projects, Health Round Table (HRT) and National Allied Health Benchmarking Consortium (NAHBC) activities and routine HNE and NSW Health reporting. As the National Allied Health Casemix Committee (NAHCC 2002, p4) states: 'Health service managers are increasingly linking inputs (e.g. staff and materials) to outputs (treated patients) and outcomes (health improvement). While many allied health professionals have comprehensive systems in place to capture the input data, little is systematically available to measure outputs.'

To address this issue, HNE Physiotherapy practitioners considered the available clinical database to be deficient. This project describes the process of identifying or developing and trialling codesets for data elements which were previously unavailable, yet vital to the data suite required to inform high-quality evaluations of practice. Three main additional data components were required to fully implement a comprehensive clinical practice evaluation process. These were physiotherapy-relevant medical diagnosis codesets, clinical priorities and clinical outcomes. The capacity to collect these data elements was found to be deficient in the HNE Allied Health Management Information System (AHMIS) (described in the following section) and other data management systems that existed at the beginning of the project. Each of these data elements, however, is vital to evaluation of physiotherapy practice:

- *Medical diagnosis codes* assist in categorising physiotherapy intervention and outcomes for comparison and benchmarking

- *Clinical priority codes* inform the triage process
- *Clinical outcome codes* enable examination of the effectiveness of service.

Summary of trials and sites

A number of trials were conducted across the following sites. Greater Newcastle Acute Hospital Network (GNAHN) is a network of three hospital sites within HNE consisting of John Hunter Hospital (JHH), Royal Newcastle Centre (RNC) and Belmont District Hospital (BDH). JHH is a 550-bed facility. It is the largest tertiary referral and teaching centre within HNE. It provides treatment for a range of specialities and services for the local community, including the only trauma centre in NSW outside Sydney. JHH emergency department is the busiest in NSW. The RNC centre has 144 beds, providing specialist services, and some medical, diagnostic and outpatient ambulatory care services. BDH is a 75-bed acute facility. Services provided include general medicine, general surgery, day surgery, coronary care unit, gynaecology, neonatal, obstetrics and a 24-hour emergency department.

In addition, two related sites joined the project. The Calvary Mater Newcastle (CMN) is a tertiary referral hospital, and has an agreement with HNE to provide a range of services including emergency care, medical, oncology and surgical, pharmacology and toxicology. It is the Hunter region's major centre for oncology services. Cessnock District Hospital (CDH) is a 61-bed acute facility. Services include general medicine, general surgery, orthopaedics, urology, gynaecology, obstetrics and a 24-hour emergency department. The trials and sites are summarised in Table 1.1.

Background

Prior data management in HNE Allied Health and Physiotherapy

In HNE, the system available for data collection and reporting consists of the Allied Health Management Information System (AHMIS) software package into which coded data is entered and extracted.

Table 1.1: Summary of trials/enquiry and sites

Data element	Trial or enquiry	Site conducted
1. Medical diagnosis codes	a. Audit of medical diagnosis codes utilised, patient count and occasions of service (OOS)	RNC
	b. The efficacy of utilising codes assigned for a previous admission or episode of care in emergency. (Target of enquiry was low back pain)	JHH and RNC
	c. Trial of draft subset of ICD-10 Codes	RNC, BDH
	d. Trial of Petersen Classification System (PCS) of Coding	RNC, Calvary Mater, Cessnock District Hospital
2. Outcome measure codes	a. Trial of AusTOMS (Australian Therapy Outcome Measures) for inpatient orthopaedics total knee replacement patients	RNC
	b. Trial of AusTOMS and Patient Specific Functional Scale (PSFS) for inpatient cardiopulmonary patients	JHH
	c. Trial of Patient Specific Functional Scale (PSFS) for antenatal outpatients	JHH
3. Clinical priority codes	Development and trial of clinical priority codes	
	a. Mapping of services and developemtn of standard codesets	a. All sites of the former Hunter Health
	b. Trial of codeset	b. GNAHN

A HNE Allied Health Data Dictionary and Codeset Reference Group was established in 2000 to coordinate the development of standardised generic and profession-specific codesets for allied health activity. The HAHS AHMIS Codeset provides a suite of definitions for these codesets. The group worked with the existing frameworks and classification systems developed by the peak allied health body, the NAHCC, as well as NSW Health existing requirements, data dictionaries and minimum datasets (Rhodes 2001).

Benchmarking

NAHCC (2003) described recommended standards for benchmarking allied health services. Recommendations have been implemented in HNE Allied Health. Physiotherapy activity data is included as part of the JHH allied health data submission to the Health Round Table (HRT) and National Allied Health Benchmarking Consortium (NAHBC). The HRT is a membership organisation which produces a number of allied health benchmarking reports and analyses for members (Health Round Table 2011). In order to participate in this benchmarking, physiotherapy conducts coding audits to ensure data entry quality and rigour.

Data reports

The following processes are available to access, link and report data for HNE Physiotherapy:

- The AHMIS and iPIMS Outpatient Module (the electronic booking system) generate reports on data entry.
- Data extracted from AHMIS is submitted for benchmarking to the HRT and NAHBC each year.
- Data extracted from AHMIS can be used to produce ad hoc reports for a variety of purposes including clinical data-mining projects.
- Data extracted from AHMIS has been uploaded into the Health Information Exchange (HIE) which acts as a data warehouse/ database. AHMIS data is combined with other data in the HIE, e.g. morbidity data for Diagnostic Related Groups (DRGs). The HIE is directly linked to the NSW Health Department HIE. Data is extracted from the HIE particularly relating to outpatient occasions of service (OOS) coded for facility, clinical area, profession and service point (Rhodes 2002).
- Reports can be generated using Business Objects as a report writing tool. The HIE will be replaced in 2011/2012 and AHMIS data at this stage is not earmarked for inclusion in the replacement version.

Specific project aims

To ensure clean and comprehensive datasets that will facilitate clinical data mining by:

- trialing codesets for medical diagnosis of clients presenting to ambulatory care outpatients
- trialing codesets for outcome measurement for services provided by a number of facilities and clinical service streams for both inpatient and ambulatory care outpatient clients
- developing and trialling a triage clinical priority tool.

Research and practice

Within the context of this practice-based research (PBR) initiative, HNE Physiotherapy decided it was no longer sufficient to utilise data only for organisational administrative reporting. Professional bodies need to demonstrate they practice at acceptable standards to clients, the organisation and NSW Health. An isolated academic theoretical perspective regarding health practice standards does not satisfy this requirement. Academic research does not translate readily into practice nor does it necessarily ask the same questions that practitioners pose about their practice (Brownson & Jones 2009; Cohen et al. 2008). At this time, physiotherapy research linking evidence to clinical presentations is limited while concurrently there is a gap in professional literature representing the unpublished innovations of evidence-informed practice. This impedes the professional health community sharing, seeding, and growing innovative models of care generated by practice-based enquiry and based on practice wisdom. This reality makes it essential to evaluate and publish what is actually happening 'on the ground' or 'at the coalface' of clinical service delivery. It is important for a learning organisation to support practitioner researchers to assess clinical health service delivery.

In social work and allied health, academics, rather than practitioners, predominantly write for publication thereby advancing the professional knowledge base and their professional careers (Hutson & Lichtiger 2002). However, in the current context, practitioners and practice managers have a role to contribute to the body of professional knowledge. Kirk (1999, p303) states: 'the research literature is itself fragmented, of uneven and questionable quality, and not very user-friendly anyway'. At this time, practitioner and practice manager enquiry into individual and programmatic clinical practice carries a dual benefit of facilitating application of enhanced practice-based wisdom, and an overall culture of service excellence and ongoing improvement. In undertaking this task, practitioners and practice managers have an opportunity to access the database of information collected for clinical and organisational reporting. This data can be utilised as a valuable source for exploring and cross-tabulating clinical relationships and subsequent reflection. Evidence-informed learning can then be systematically applied to individual and programmatic practice innovation in an ongoing improvement cycle.

If practice guidelines recommended by researchers are not validated by practice and practitioners, their utility is limited. Their practical application to diverse presentations and demographics cannot be refined. The service provider has responsibility for the service they provide, and to make the judgements regarding interventions for their clients. A complementary relationship between clinical practice and research is advised to maximise the quality of service to clients, and utility of research-based guidelines (Hutson & Lichtiger 2002). To achieve these service benefits, practice managers with the assistance of practitioners need to establish a culture and processes to support these activities which are applicable in the clinic environment.

Writing about adolescent health and mental health, Peake, Epstein, Mirabito and Surko (2004) state that the specific characteristics of practice-based research (PBR) tools and research-based practice (RBP) tools differ. They suggest models whereby practice-based research and research-based practice are considered as a continuum. Data generated can be 'aggregated and analysed' to provide the basis 'for staff reflection and program change' in a similar way as reported by Peake et al. (2004, p56).

Applying this to HNE Physiotherapy, an organisational development goal was to provide the opportunity to form the physiotherapy workforce into what Peake et al. (2004, p58) described as 'A Practice-Based Research Group'. This group could apply practice-based research (PBR) and research-based practice (RBP) methodology to clinical inquiry, and clinical service or program improvement. The process aimed to empower the workforce to contribute to physiotherapy program management and improvement, and a culture of service excellence. The flexibility afforded by this approach renders it particularly beneficial in a climate of ongoing organisational change.

Research methodology

The overall task of refining existing and developing new data codesets was complicated. Here action research principles were found to be valuable in implementing a management strategy to achieve the goals of this project, one that took place with a large team operating in a complex 'real life' non-static environment. Reason and Bradbury (2001) describe action research as an interactive enquiry process that balances problem solving actions implemented in a collaborative context with data-driven collaborative analysis or research to understand underlying causes, enabling future predictions about personal and organisational change. It is a useful management strategy to drive a process for achieving whole-of-organisation goals over time in a changing environment (Reil 2010).

Susman (1983) distinguishes five phases to be conducted within each research cycle. These steps continue until the problem is solved. These cycles of reflection and new action are shown to be useful where it is not possible or relevant to implement one academically sound but rigid study or randomised controlled trial (RCT) (McNiff 2000). The nature of the problem, resources and personnel involved, theory of practice, organisational needs, infrastructure etc. can all change over time, rendering an initial study design outdated. Alternately, a number of achievable and realistic smaller trials can be linked to build toward a goal and service improvement incrementally. The design of each component trial may have limitations due to it being one of pragmatic convenience in the busy clinical environment; however, some degree of rigour can be achieved by relentlessly applying the process over time.

Clinical data mining

Another purpose of this research project was to utilise valid data for practice research projects to improve clinical practices and service delivery. There are impediments to achieving this in the busy clinic environment. However, with the assistance of Irwin Epstein, HNE Physiotherapy has applied clinical data-mining (CDM) principles and processes in clinic to support practice-based enquiry (Epstein 2010). Data-mining methodology is limited in its capacity to inform causal relationships. Hence the practice evidence informed by these tools is qualified.

The process

A team of physiotherapy managers and practitioners reviewed the codesets available, and determined those to be implemented or developed. Trials were conducted as outlined in Table 1.1. Reliability of the tool was established in the trial of the Petersen Classification System (PCS) (Petersen et al. 2003; Petersen et al. 2004) as described in Chapter 8. In the HNE trials of outcome and priority codesets, reliability was established through practice-based consistency agreements. Face validity of tools was judged by senior clinicians, e.g. selection of the PCS for coding medical diagnosis in a pathoanatomic model.

Uniform methods of data management and entry were developed to promote standard processes: a) a manual was developed to guide use of the iPIMS Outpatient Module electronic booking system as a service management tool to assist with appropriate responsiveness to clinical priority; b) staff were trained in PCS; and c) regular activity data coding audits were conducted, the results of which were actioned by departmental delegates.

Literature review

A review of literature relevant to physiotherapy practice databases was then undertaken. This literature provides a foundation for physiotherapy to refine and develop codesets applicable to practice and valid for data mining. However, no literature was located defining a process for this vital locally based but nationally relevant codeset development. Many of the codesets discussed are cumbersome and not easily applied at a local level. Nevertheless, the history and process of codeset development reveals a broad range of themes vital for both background and guidance for this complex task.

Classifications for medical diagnosis

Medical diagnosis codes for ambulatory care outpatient physiotherapy clients have application for categorising physiotherapy activity to facilitate data analysis of interventions and treatment outcomes. There is some concordance between the medical diagnosis, the indicator for intervention or therapy diagnosis code (NAHCC 2000). There are a number of codesets available for medical diagnoses which have inherent benefits and limitations when utilised to categorise HNE Physiotherapy activity data. A number of these are explored below.

The International Classification of Diseases (ICD)

The International Classification of Diseases (ICD) is a detailed description of known diseases and injuries. It is published by the World Health Organization (WHO) and is used worldwide for morbidity and mortality statistics. A medical condition and disease (or group of related diseases) is described with its diagnosis and given a unique ICD code for diagnosis or procedure. These are to be replaced by International Classification of Diseases-10-Clinical Modification (ICD-10-CM), for diagnosis codes, and International Classification of Diseases-10-Procedure Coding System (ICD-10-PCS), for procedure codes (World Health Organization 2011). NAHCC (2002) report allied health sensitive codes from the International Classification of Diseases-10-Australian Modification (ICD-10-AM) third edition. The list has been identified as useful to professional activities and interventions.

Having widespread application worldwide and particularly in Australian public health, the ICD-10 codeset has clear benefits for utilisation as a coding tool. It permits creation of a database which can be utilised to compare activity between organisations. However, the ICD-10 codeset is not sensitive enough to code some of the clinical diagnosis hypotheses used by physiotherapy practitioners. (The medical diagnostic codes available in HNE AHMIS are from ICD-9 to date but could be mapped to ICD-10-AM codes).

Diagnostic Related Group (DRG)

Diagnostic Related Groups (DRGs) are a classification system used in a casemix funding model. The classification system is used to group in-patient stays into clinically meaningful categories of similar levels of complexity that consume similar amounts of resources. Allocation of an Australian refined diagnostic related group (AR-DRG) involves a pre-scribed process whereby one acute inpatient episode of care is allocated to one AR-DRG (Royal Children's Hospital Melbourne 2010).

The HRT process reports of inpatient activity against DRGs to facilitate benchmarking and practice review of inpatients. However, processes to effectively manage physiotherapy ambulatory care outpatient data needs to be established.

International Classification of Function (ICF)

Functioning and disability associated with health conditions can be classified using the Diagnostic Related Groups, Disabilities and Health Short Version (ICF) developed by the WHO (World Health Organization 2001). Three components are classified in ICF: body functions and structures, activities and participation, and environmental factors.

Unfortunately, the ICF was considered by HNE Physiotherapy to be too cumbersome a tool to apply in the busy clinic without considerable development of processes to support its use. It has not been widely applied and reported for comparisons between organisations, or in the clinical practice literature.

Indicators for Intervention (IFI)

Indicators for Intervention (IFI) were developed by the NAHCC (Australian Psychological Society Ltd 2008) using the ICF codes to provide information on the reason why the allied health professional was providing care to the client, e.g. the symptoms, behaviour or circumstances. IFIs have a classification structure that drills down to more specific IFIs.

The IFIs at the D level are very similar to or identical to ICD-10-AM codes. It is postulated that this provides for the possibility of mapping across classifications based on ICD.

The IFI classification has been used as the source of the local codeset for Therapy Diagnosis in the HNE data dictionary. For physiotherapy purposes, the IFI, however, does not capture adequately the patient's presenting issue and cannot utilised effectively in place of a medical diagnosis code for clinical practice evaluation.

Clinical coding

Low back pain (LBP) has been the target of investigation in HNE Physiotherapy CDM trials. Clinical research literature has reported a number of attempts to classify LBP based on pathoanatomic criteria. Reports indicated that the prevalence of non-specific low back pain (NSLBP) as essentially undiagnosed LBP is 85% of LBP presentations (Waddell 2004). For coding purposes in the physiotherapy clinic, therefore, ICD-10 coding for LBP would largely default to one code – M54.5 (LBP). However, some reports indicated that specific subgroups of presentations of NSLBP which received intervention specific to the hypothesised subgroup had a larger treatment effect or better outcome (Kent & Keating 2004). As a result, pathoanatomic models of coding for LBP were being reported. The PCS (Petersen et al. 2003; Petersen et al. 2004) appeared to have face validity and acceptable reliability for coding pathoanatomic subclassifications of LBP.

More recent literature has moved away from pathoanatomic classifications of low back pain as a useful tool to assist clinical management and improve patient outcomes. Statistical prediction models for spinal pain treatment decision-making have been developed and reported (Beneciuk et al. 2009; May & Rosedale 2009; Stanton et al. 2010).

Classifications for outcomes

Outcome measurement is important for organisational practice evaluation and in the successful application of evidence to practice in the clinical situation. The reasoning process in treatment decision-making involves the continuous, judicious assessment and re-evaluation of patient outcomes throughout the clinical interaction. Clinical decision-making in physiotherapy is multidimensional. To apply evidence to clinical practice, physiotherapy clinical decision-making integrates the available body of evidence with the presenting clinical situation in cognitively based rational models of reasoning (Edwards et al. 2004) and meaning-based forms of reasoning (Cohen et al. 2008). In recent years, physiotherapy literature has reported the development and clinical application of tools that aim to facilitate clinical selection of interventions for given presentations which have been demonstrated to have an increased probability of favourable response (Brennan et al. 2006; Fritz et al. 2003; Long et al. 2004). Randomised controlled trials (RCT) have demonstrated the improved efficacy of intervention selection based upon specific clinical presentations that are predictive of a favourable response (Brennan et al. 2006; Fritz et al. 2003; Long et al. 2004). However, the body of knowledge reported to date in this respect is limited. Under these circumstances, the reliance on rational hypothetico-deductive reasoning increases, and therefore the reliance on outcome measures to inform this process.

A number of outcome measures were reviewed. Most were reliable and valid but only for specific clinical conditions. Whilst invaluable in specific practice evaluation, their merit in larger organisation-wide practice evaluation was limited. In contrast, the AusTOMs (Perry et al. 2004) and Patient Specific Functional Scale (PSFS) (Stratford et al. 1995) outcome tools appeared to provide some capacity to apply reliable and valid tools on an organisational level to evaluate practice outcomes.

AusTOMs (Perry et al. 2004)

The AusTOMs outcome measure tools aimed to provide a measure of therapy outcomes for physiotherapy, speech pathology and occupational therapy. There are nine AusTOMs scales for physiotherapy to apply across different clinical caseloads. Each of the AusTOMs for physiotherapy scales has four domains: impairment, activity limitation, participation restriction and wellbeing.

AusTOMS appeared to provide a number of potential benefits as outcome measures for HNE Physiotherapy. The AusTOMs for physiotherapy scale headings are based on the WHO ICF body functions and structures. Australian physiotherapists considered it important to have one underlying concept on which all the AusTOMs card headings would be based. Additionally, NAHCC (2002) recommended AusTOMs as a data system which might be required for successful management of allied health services in acute care facilities. Validity and reliability had also been addressed by the team developing the measures.

The Patient Specific Functional Scale (PSFS)

The Patient Specific Functional Scale (PSFS) (Stratford et al. 1995) is a patient-specific outcome measure which investigates functional status. Patients are asked to select up to five activities with which they have difficulty due to their condition. They are asked to rate the functional limitation experienced with these activities. The PSFS is intended to be used in conjunction with condition-specific measures (Stratford et al. 1995).

Classifications for priority

Clinical priority is usually assigned to a clinical presentation based upon clinical need, urgency and risk of adversity. Organisational re-quirements to support the whole client population strategically are also often embedded in priority statements, e.g. clients awaiting discharge are often afforded priority if other clients require admission to support 'patient flows'. Clinical priority can be assigned at triage, priority state-ments are often accompanied by recommended timeframes for service. A number of clinical prioritisation tools have been shared through the HRT and NAHBC. These priority tools are often locally applicable. Local service mapping and reference to evidence regarding target ser-vice timeframes is utilised to develop tools specific to the local service.

Cleaning up the codes 1: medical diagnosis code

Problem

From the initial AHMIS implementation, there were 83 pages or 1583 ICD-9 medical diagnosis codes in the Physiotherapy Data Dictionary. Physiotherapy reported that the codeset was too large and inconsistently constructed to capture reliable and valid data for service and clinical evaluation. Medical diagnosis can be captured for clients who are inpatients as AHMIS data can be linked via their MRN to diagnostic coding for inpatients entered in iPM. There was no validated consistent process to allocate medical diagnosis to ambulatory care outpatient physiotherapy clients.

Aim

To identify and trial appropriate medical diagnosis codesets for conditions presenting to ambulatory care outpatient physiotherapy which would be relevant to be used for clinical and service evaluation and reporting, and data mining.

Method

HNE Physiotherapy agreed that the Greater Newcastle Acute Hospital Network (GNAHN) (which consists of John Hunter Hospital, Royal Newcastle Centre and Belmont District Hospital) would conduct the trials.

An audit of the medical diagnosis codes assigned to ambulatory Royal Newcastle Centre (RNC) Physiotherapy clients and the frequency of their use was completed. Refer to Table 1.2 for the 10 most frequent diagnosis codes.

Of the four most common codes, low back pain (LBP) was the condition which was almost entirely managed in ambulatory care outpatients, and therefore did not have an organisationally assigned medical diagnosis. Clients presenting with LBP were chosen as a test group to develop the methodology to be applied to other clinical conditions. Clients presenting with LBP represented a high-volume service user group: 414 patients were managed through 1487 occasions of service between 1 July 2004 and 30 June 2005 (Table 1.2).

Table 1.2: RNC physiotherapy audit – 10 most frequent medical diagnosis codes and occasions of service (OOS)

Diagnosis code	Descriptor	Patient count	Frequency OOS
81.54	Knee: total knee replacement	911	4344
81.51	Hip: THR	559	2055
820	Hip: neck of femur	240	1527
724.2	L/S: low back pain	358	1251
82.4	Hand: suture of muscle tendon and fascia	190	775
723.1	C/S: neck pain	183	683
719.46	Knee: joint pain	199	573
726.1	Shoulder: rotator cuff lesion/ incom tear	119	533
82	Hand: OPS on muscle tendon and fascia	137	476
813.42	Wrist: radius-distal end	172	427

Physiotherapy proposed to evaluate the following codesets for application in HNE:

a. ICD-10 (initially ICD-9) codesets for diagnosis and procedure

b. the Petersen Classification System (PCS).

ICD-10 codesets for diagnosis and procedure

For a presentation to ambulatory care outpatient physiotherapy related to a prior related admission or attendance at emergency, a medical diagnosis code would have been assigned by the organisation.

i) Continuum of care: clients presenting post a related admission or attendance at emergency

Physiotherapy initially aimed to ensure codes assigned to ambulatory care outpatients presenting with LBP would be consistent with ICD-10 diagnosis and procedure codes assigned for previous related admissions or attendance at emergency. It was hypothesised that data could be linked if the same codes were used. It was also hypothesised that different medical diagnosis codes entered in allied health data fields may cause data corruption in the HIE. Physiotherapy proposed to review diagnosis and procedure codes assigned to these clients by hospital and Emergency Department (ED) coders. This situation would apply to the two following client groups:

Presentations following a related preceding inpatient admission

To evaluate the efficacy of utilising ICD-10 codes assigned for a previous related admission, physiotherapy consulted the Clinical Information Department regarding selection of the prime diagnosis or procedure code. At the time of consultation, coder's advice was that there were a multitude of codes applied for one admission, and selection of a single prime code which would be most relevant to the physiotherapy presentation would be difficult.

Presentations following a related preceding attendance in emergency

To evaluate the efficacy of utilising codes assigned for a previous related episode of care in emergency with LBP, physiotherapy conducted a CDM study of clients presenting to emergency.

Method

Data was collected retrospectively for all patients presenting to ED at JHH with a soft tissue injury (STI) over a three-month period in 2007. Data was also collected for all patients treated by physiotherapy in the ED for any clinical condition.

Participants

During the period of the study, there were 777 patients with STI who presented to the ED. A total of 227 patients were referred to physiotherapy during this period. From the total presenting to ED with STI, 55 were referred to outpatient ambulatory care physiotherapy. Twenty-eight of these presented with LBP.

CDM findings

The total number of presentations to the ED during the period was 15,142. The most frequent referrals to physiotherapy were received for falls management. This constituted 54.6% of all referrals to physiotherapy. Correspondingly, the most common physiotherapy intervention applied was mobility assessment. Mobility assessment constituted 71.4% of all physiotherapy interventions. Of all STIs presenting to ED, 7.1% were referred to physiotherapy in ED. Of these STIs referred to physiotherapy in ED, 50.9% were for LBP, and 39% of these were subsequently referred to outpatient physiotherapy.

Discussion

The results of this audit indicate that the primary role of physiotherapy is to perform mobility assessments. STI management is a minor role of physiotherapy in the ED.

Conclusion

The limited number of clients presenting to emergency with LBP and referred to outpatient physiotherapy has been noted. The process of extracting the clinical information to complete the process was extremely labour-intensive. Consideration of the value of utilising the code assigned by ED in light of this is in progress.

ii) Clients referred with LBP unrelated to a previous admission or attendance at emergency

Physiotherapy conducted two data-mining trials to investigate codesets for LBP and their capacity to be utilised to evaluate clinical practice. The two codesets trialled were the ICD-10 and Petersen Classification System (PCS).

a) ICD-10 codes

A subset of potential ICD-10 codes for clients presenting to ambulatory care outpatients physiotherapy without a previous related admission or attendance at emergency was drafted. The ICD-10 subset of codes was based on clinical practice guidelines for LBP and recommendations regarding categories for triage, i.e. non-specific low back pain (NSLBP), radiculopathy and specific LBP (Clinical Standards Advisory Group 1994; Koes et al. 2001). Detailed results of the trial are reported in Chapter 8. Refer to Table 1.3 for draft ICD-10 codes for LBP.

Table 1.3: Proposed ICD-10 medical diagnosis codes for outpatients musculoskeletal physiotherapy

LBP type	Code description	ICD-10 code
Non-specific LBP		M54.5
Radiculopathy	No evidence of IV disc disorder	M54.1
	Evidence of IV disc disorder	M51.1
Specific LBP	Spinal stenosis	M48.0
	Spondylolisthesis/ Spondylolysis	M53.2
	Ankylosing spondylitis	M45
	Fracture – Lx	S32.0
	Fracture – Sx	S32.1
	Fracture – coccyx	S32.2
	Infection	M46.4
	Cancer	C80
	SC compression	G95.2
	CE syndrome	G83.4

b) Pathoanatomic classification of LBP: the PCS

The Petersen Classification System (PCS) was consequently trialled by physiotherapy in 2005 (Petersen et al. 2004). Detailed results of the trial are reported in Chapter 8.

Limitation of the Petersen coding trial

NSW Health employs coders to apply ICD-10 and assign DRGs. Physiotherapy has not been trained in coding of ICD-10. It is possible that coders would have coded the client population differently. The ICD-10 codeset available to staff on the AHMIS package was not limited to the subset of codes chosen for the trial. As physiotherapy academic enquiry has developed, there has been a move away from pathoanatomic classifications.

Discussion

Both codesets trialled were able to be utilised to mine clinical data, and gave consistent reports for a large number of clinical parameters (refer to Chapter 8).

ICD-10 is a widely applied codeset in public health. For routine data collection, the ICD-10 codeset may have advantages over the Peterson Classification System if its utilisation can facilitate comparison or benchmarking of data. However, the Petersen Classification System (PCS) may have advantages for specific coding for prospective trials aiming to investigate pathoanatomic clinical questions.

More recently reported statistical prediction models for spinal pain treatment decision-making (Beneciuk et al. 2009; May & Rosedale 2009; Stanton et al. 2010) may have implications for future trials in HNE.

Conclusion

The ICD-10 codes in Table 1.3 will be loaded onto AHMIS based on the results of the clinical trials and enquiry to date.

Cleaning up codes 2: outcomes data

Aim/problem

This trial was conducted in the RNC. RNC outpatient physiotherapy has a long history of outcome measurement. However, for other physiotherapy clinical caseloads, outcome measurement is not as routinely applied. Current clinical guidelines recommend the use of valid and reliable outcome measures to show objective change over time that may be related to treatment. To comply, physiotherapy aimed to trial and implement outcome measures which provided sensitivity to specific clinical conditions and which were practical to apply as ongoing routine data collections. Physiotherapy also aimed to investigate if any outcome measures may have the additional benefit of being applicable across services and clinical streams to provide a capacity to measure outcomes on a larger organisational basis.

The trial aimed to investigate the use of AusTOMs and the PSFS as outcome measures within physiotherapy for specific clinical caseloads, and also across services. The tools were applied in this trial to musculoskeletal, cardiopulmonary, and women's health caseloads.

Method/action

A range of clinical specialties across GNAHN Physiotherapy undertook to trial the use of AusTOMs and the PSFS over a three-month period in 2005. Data was collected for the following samples of convenience:

a. AusTOMs was trialled for inpatient orthopaedics clients who had undergone a total knee replacement (TKR).

b. AusTOMs and the PSFS were trialled for inpatient cardiopulmonary physiotherapy.

c. The PSFS was trialled as an outcome measure for the physiotherapy treatment of antenatal outpatients referred for pelvic/back pain.

Results

a. AusTOMs were applied to inpatient orthopaedics clients who had undergone a TKR.

For patients who had undergone TKR, the average of totalled AusTOMs scores for the sample in each domain improved day 1 to day 3 and again improved at discharge.

b. AusTOMs and the PSFS were trialled for inpatient cardiopulmonary physiotherapy.

Data for initial assessment of cardiopulmonary clients for both the Aus-TOMs and PSFS was collected. The AusTOMs score and the PSFS did not correlate for this group.

c. The PSFS was trialled as an outcome measure for the physiotherapy treatment of antenatal outpatients referred for pelvic/back pain.

The measures were collected for 13 antenatal outpatients referred for pelvic/LBP. For antenatal outpatients referred for pelvic/LBP, nine participants had improved PSFS scores that indicated decreasing difficulty in performing the activities on their second physiotherapy session. Four participants had scores which indicated increased difficulty in performing the activities on their second physiotherapy session. However, the change in scores was generally only a 1–2 point difference, whereas changes of two points are considered clinically meaningful (Stratford et al. 1995). It was also noted that these four participants were all 37+ weeks gestation. Overall, 70% of the participants indicated an improvement in the ability to perform the activities of daily living (ADL) at their second physiotherapy session.

Limitations

It was initially planned for each clinical stream to trial both the PSFS and AusTOMs measure on both inpatients and outpatients (if relevant to their service). The realities of a busy clinic limited the scope of the trial, and limited the sample size.

Conclusions

a. AusTOMs were applied to inpatient orthopaedics clients who had undergone a TKR.

AusTOMs was a cumbersome tool, especially to apply all domains as recommended, and not appropriate for some patient groups such as acute TKRs where improvement of impairment and disability is expected over time.

b. AusTOMs and the PSFS were trialled for inpatient cardiopulmonary physiotherapy.

The AusTOMs and PSFS measures did not correlate for cardiopulmonary inpatients. The AusTOMs was cumbersome for inpatient use. It was postulated that a more clinically sensitive measure for cardiopulmonary clients than both the AusTOMs and PSFS may need to be trialled.

c. The PSFS was trialled as an outcome measure for the physiotherapy treatment of antenatal outpatients referred for pelvic/back pain.

Physiotherapists found the use of the PSFS measure to be easy to use and time effective for antenatal pelvic/back pain patients. It also appeared that physiotherapy intervention for these patients was generally effective in improving their ability to perform ADL.

Overall

The PSFS was found to be a more helpful tool and will continue to be used for GNAHN Physiotherapy ambulatory care musculoskeletal outpatients and antenatal pelvic and LBP clients as appropriate.

Other clinical streams will investigate the use of appropriate valid and reliable outcome measures that are pertinent to the conditions they manage.

Cleaning up codes 3: clinical priorities

Trial 1: Managing ambulatory care outpatient clinical priorities

Background

Ambulatory care outpatient data for wait time from referral to intervention was routinely entered by physiotherapy staff of some HNE departments, from 2001. Data was reported monthly and compared to targets to provide an indicator for client access to service.

Problem

Wait-time data collected and reported from the facilities of GNAHN indicated cross-department wait-time discrepancies. Anecdotally, physiotherapists in GNAHN and across HNE reported that patients had registered on numerous department wait lists for service in order to obtain a physiotherapy service with the smallest wait time. Additionally, patients registered on wait lists for department services of their preference, not necessarily related to the clinical specialty offered by the service for the condition for which they required intervention. This practice meant that wait-time data for a facility could not be utilised as a true indication of service need and consequently need to redeploy resources responsively.

iPM Outpatient Module was introduced in GNAHN Physiotherapy in 2005 to provide an electronic process to book ambulatory care outpatient appointments.

Aim

- To map HNE Physiotherapy ambulatory care outpatient services
- to document agreed triage clinical priorities for ambulatory outpatient services
- to document wait-time targets for service delivery
- to implement iPM Outpatient Module to operate as a service management tool to address the wait-list issue in GNAHN Physiotherapy.

Method

1. Physiotherapy conducted a HNE-wide process to map outpatient services, document agreed triage clinical priorities for ambulatory outpatient services, and wait-time targets for service delivery.

2. iPIMS was implemented to create a cross-facility/department waiting list which could be viewed by managers at any time during the month.

3. Data audits of iPM Outpatient Module and AHMIS were conducted to establish reliability.

4. Processes and a manual were developed to support the use of iPM Outpatient Module as a tool to assist service management of wait lists (i.e. wait times, clinical triage priorities and available appointments in clinics across GNAHN Physiotherapy facility departments could be managed to offer a client the most appropriate and timely appointment for their condition).

5. A monthly report detailing activity and waiting times was established.

6. If waiting times for outpatient physiotherapy were not within target for priority, strategies to manage those patients whose wait for

service exceeds target were discussed and implemented. Strategies included:

a. redistributing staff across clinical areas
b. re-prioritising duties
c. offering patients appointments at other sites
d. implementing 'assessment days' to triage the waiting list.

Results

The triage priority codes for ambulatory care outpatient services are documented in Table 1.4.

Data indicated improved access to outpatient physiotherapy, e.g. at BDH the waiting list for outpatients physiotherapy decreased from 109 to 40 by December 2004. These wait times were largely within target by May 2005.

Conclusion

The process was successful in managing the ambulatory care outpatient wait list.

What has changed?

For patients

Medical diagnosis

Some reports indicate that specific subgroups of presentations of NSLBP which receive intervention specific to the hypothesised subgroup had a larger treatment effect or better outcome. Therefore, implementation of a process to code for LBP clinical diagnosis may have assisted the HNE.

Physiotherapy clinician's reasoning process to match the intervention with the highest probability of a favourable outcome to the presentation was improved. This may have assisted HNE Physiotherapy to achieve the service results reported in Chapter 8. Evaluation of the data describing clinical management of LBP in Chapter 8 indicates management largely conforming to published standards in some key areas.

Table 1.4: iPM triage priority codes for physiotherapy

Priority Code	Priority Type	Description (examples)	Target
Walk-ins	Walk-in	Appointment offered on same day, e.g. fit crutches from clinic	0 days
Priority 1	Acute	- Condition less than 6 weeks	1 week
		- Hand Injury	
		- Post-operative	
		- Following removal of plaster (may be walk-in)	
		- For a mobility assessment	
		- Unable to self-care safely and adequately	
		- Primary carer for someone disabled	
		- Off work/school because of condition	
Priority 2	Sub-acute	- Condition 6 weeks to 3 months	3 weeks
Priority 7	Chronic	- Conditions greater than 3 months that are stable, i.e. no neurological symptoms or severe exacerbation	6 weeks
Priority 9	Awaiting treatment	- Unavailable for treatment	
		- Treatment postponed for medical reasons	

Outcome measures

In the absence of a comprehensive body of knowledge regarding clinical prediction rules, deductive reasoning is an important element of clinical management. Outcome measurement is important in the successful application of evidence to clinical practice and applying deductive reasoning. As such, outcome measurement is an important element of clinical management and service evaluation. Wider introduction of outcome measurement across physiotherapy services could be expected to have contributed to improved client management.

Clinical priority

Introduction of clinical priority coding and processes to review data and scheduling appears to be related to improved service responsiveness to client need. GNAHN ambulatory care outpatient wait times for service have improved, and are generally within target timeframes.

Team, practice, organisational and research benefits

a. Practitioners and programs practice informed by data linking evidence and practice

Practitioners and program managers have more data management tools to link research and practice as a basis of reflection. Specific practice and program benefits have been described in Chapter 8.

b. Physiotherapy workforce culture of excellence: linking evidence, practice, empirical data and ongoing practice improvement

All clinical teams in GNAHN Physiotherapy have been involved in this program of projects. The process has encouraged a culture of total quality management in staff which contributes to excellence in service. Practitioners and program managers have embedded a method to apply research-based practice (RBP) and practice-based research (PBR). The process has helped inform key staff about data-mining methodology and assisted seed projects which have had positive client effects

c. Research tools to drive practice, program and organisational change systematically over time in a busy clinical environment.

The action research and data-mining tools have been applied to drive practitioner, program and organisational physiotherapy service change over time in a complex, changing and challenging clinical environment. Empowering practitioners as researchers has enabled HNE Physiotherapy to operate as a 'learning organisation'.

d. Practitioner researchers to inform the professional community and body of knowledge

The relative lack of professional published knowledge relating practitioner- or program-based enquiry diminishes the capacity to directly apply evidence to practice and result in true clinical and service improvement. The processes applied in this program and medley of projects have attempted to commence redressing this gap.

Conclusion

The codesets and processes developed, implemented and trialled for medical diagnosis, clinical priority, and outcome (clinical and service) are tools which have been utilised to link data and inform both research and practice.

Implementation of these tools with the practice-based research methodologies was applied to drive organisational development processes over time. These have resulted in a number of practice and organisational improvements and benefits. The physiotherapy workforce is being empowered with tools and a culture of inquiry and excellence to investigate and improve their practice. They in turn can contribute to physiotherapy program and organisational initiatives to drive improvement informed by data generated by practice linked with research methodologies. In addition, they may contribute to further knowledge development for physiotherapy in general that is informed by practice and initiated by practitioners.

Acknowledgements

The project team and authorship is large, representing the widespread contribution of Hunter New England Health and Greater Newcastle Acute Hospital Network (John Hunter Hospital, Royal Newcastle Centre and Belmont District Hospital) physiotherapy and other discipline staff. The contribution of all staff and partners is acknowledged and greatly appreciated: Natalie Walsh, Emma Mitchell, Kieren Brown, Veronica Parraga, Tim Lee, Mary Caine, Peter Osmotherly, Suzanne Snodgrass, Matthew Bryant, Carla Dyson, other members of the Physiotherapy Data Dictionary Working Party, Physiotherapy Greater Newcastle Acute Hospital Network Ambulatory Care/iPM Implementation Working Party, Physiotherapy Research Interest Group, and all Greater Newcastle Acute Hospital Network and Hunter New England

Health physiotherapy staff who contributed, supported teams and collected data.

References

Australian Physiotherapy Council (2006). Australian standards for physiotherapy. [Online]. Available: www.physiocouncil.com.au/Australian%20Standards%20 for%20Physiotherapy/ [Accessed 25 March 2011].

Beneciuk JM, Bishop MD & George SZ (2009). Clinical prediction rules for physical therapy interventions: a systematic review. *Physical Therapy*, 89(2): 114–24.

Brennan GP, Fritz JM, Hunter SJ, Thackeray A, Delitto A & Erhard RE (2006). Identifying subgroups of patients with acute/subacute 'nonspecific' low back pain: results of a randomized clinical trial. *Spine*, 31(6): 623–31.

Brownson RC & Jones E (2009). Bridging the gap: translating research into policy and practice. *Preventive Medicine*, 49(4): 313–15.

Clinical Standards Advisory Group (1994). *Back pain*. London: HMSO.

Cohen DJ, Crabtree BF, Etz RS, Balasubramanian BA, Donahue KE, Leviton LC, Clark EC, Isaacson NF, Stange KC & Green LW (2008). Fidelity versus flexibility: translating evidence-based research into practice. *American Journal of Preventive Medicine*, 35(5 Suppl.): S381–S389.

Edwards I, Jones M, Carr J, Braunack-Mayer A & Jensen GM (2004). Clinical reasoning strategies in physical therapy. *Physical Therapy*, 84(4): 312–30; discussion 331–15.

Epstein I (2010). *Clinical data-mining: integrating practice and research*. New York: Oxford University Press.

Fritz JM, Delitto A & Erhard RE (2003). Comparison of classification-based physical therapy with therapy based on clinical practice guidelines for patients with acute low back pain: a randomized clinical trial. *Spine*, 28(13): 1363–71; discussion 1372.

Guyatt G, Haynes B, Jaeschke R, Meade M, Wilson M, Montori V & Richardson S (2008). The philosophy of evidence-based medicine. In G Guyatt, D Rennie,

M Meade & D Cook (Eds). *Users' guides to the medical literature: a manual for evidence-based clinical practice* (pp5-16). 2nd edn. USA: McGraw Hill Medical.

Health Round Table (2011). Compare performance: allied health. [Online]. Available: www.healthroundtable.org/ComparePerformance/AlliedHealth/ tabid/99/Default.aspx [Accessed 25 March 2011].

Hutson C & Lichtiger E (2002). Mining clinical information in the utilization of social services. *Social Work in Health Care,* 33(3): 153-61.

Kent P & Keating J (2004). Do primary-care clinicians think that nonspecific low back pain is one condition? *Spine,* 29(9): 1022-31.

Kirk SA (1999). Good intentions are not enough: practice guidelines for social work. *Research on Social Work Practice,* 9(3): 302-10.

Koes BW, van Tulder MW, Ostelo R, Kim Burton A & Waddell G (2001). Clinical guidelines for the management of low back pain in primary care: an international comparison. *Spine,* 26(22), 2504-13; discussion 2513-2504.

Long A, Donelson R & Fung T (2004). Does it matter which exercise? A randomized control trial of exercise for low back pain. *Spine,* 29(23): 2593-602.

May S & Rosedale R (2009). Prescriptive clinical prediction rules in back pain research: a systematic review. *Journal of Manual and Manipulative Therapy,* 17(1): 36-45.

McNiff J (2000). *Action research in organisations.* London: Routledge.

National Allied Health Casemix Committee (2003). Standards for benchmarking allied health services. April.

National Allied Health Casemix Committee (2002). National allied health casemix committee data manual v1 May.

National Allied Health Casemix Committee (2000). Report on the development of allied health indicators for intervention (IFI) and performance indicators (PI) and revision of allied health-sensitive ICD-10-AM codes for inclusion in ICD-10-AM Edition Two.

National Centre for Classification in Health (2002). ICD-10-AM. 3rd edn, July. Available at: www.nahcc.org.au/review.htm [Accessed on 5 July 2011].

Peake K, Epstein I, Mirabito D & Surko M (2004). Development and utilization of a practice-based, adolescent intake questionnaire (adquest): surveying which risks, worries, and concerns urban youth want to talk about. *Social Work in Mental Health*, 3(1–2): 55–82.

Perry A, Morris M, Unsworth C, Duckett S, Skeat J, Dodd K, Taylor N & Reilly K (2004). Therapy outcome measures for allied health practitioners in Australia: the AusTOMs. *International Journal for Quality in Health Care*, 16(4): 285–91.

Petersen T, Laslett M, Thorsen H, Manniche C, Ekdahl C & Jacobsen S (2003). Diagnostic classification of non-specific low back pain. a new system integrating patho-anatomic and clinical categories. *Physiotherapy Theory and Practice*, 19(4): 213–37.

Petersen T, Olsen S, Laslett M, Thorsen H, Manniche C, Ekdahl C & Jacobsen S (2004). Inter-tester reliability of a new diagnostic classification system for patients with non-specific low back pain. *Australian Journal of Physiotherapy*, 50(2): 85–94.

Reason P & Bradbury H (2001). *Handbook of action research: participative inquiry and practice*. London: Sage.

Reil M (2010). Understanding action research. Centre for Collaborative Action Research. Pepperdine University. [Online]. Available: cadres.pepperdine.edu/ccar/define.html [Accessed 25 March 2011].

Rhodes D (2002). Allied health management information system reports analysis: Hunter Health.

Rhodes D (2001). Allied health management information system codeset: Hunter Health.

Royal Children's Hospital Melbourne (2010). Diagnostic related groups classification system. [Online]. Available: www.rch.org.au/rchhis/coding/index.cfm?doc_id=12153 [Accessed 25 March 2011].

Stanton TR, Hancock MJ, Maher CG & Koes BW (2010). Critical appraisal of clinical prediction rules that aim to optimize treatment selection for musculoskeletal conditions. *Physical Therapy*, 90(6): 843–54.

Stratford P, Gill C, Westaway M & Binkley J (1995). Assessing disability and change on individual patients: a report of a patient specific measure. *Physiotherapy Canada*, 47(4): 258–63.

Susman GI (1983). Action research: a sociotechnical systems perspective. In Morgan G (Ed). *Beyond method: strategies for social research* (pp95–113). London: Sage Publications.

The Australian Psychological Society Ltd (2008). *Indicators for intervention (IFI) project.* Melbourne: The Australian Psychological Society Ltd.

Waddell G (2004). *The back pain revolution.* 2nd edn. Edinburgh: Churchill Livingstone.

World Health Organization (2011). International classification of diseases. Geneva. [Online]. Available: www.who.int/classifications/icd/en/ [Accessed 25 March 2011].

World Health Organization (2001). International classification of functioning, disability and health, short version. Geneva. [Online]. Available: www.who.int/classifications/icf/en/ [Accessed 25 March 2011].

Chapter 2

The long and winding road: creating an outcome tool for 'prospective data mining' of social work services

Fran Hodgson and Roslyn Giles

Spurred on by contemporary health service accountability demands for evidence of effectiveness and demonstrable practice outcomes, a small, changing band of social workers set out on a path to develop a client-focused outcome tool for social work health practice and a new source of data for mining. Findings to date reveal encouraging information about client experiences of health social workers' practice and challenging implications for future practice-based research.

Key words: social work outcomes, client-focused outcomes, research

In many health settings, social work clinicians record client-related activity information into some form of administrative data program. In addition to demographic information on age, gender and location, these programs generate information that describes activity; for example, how many clients have been seen, what interventions were used over what timeframe and with what frequency. Social workers also complete assessments with clients about their family dynamics, social networks, financial stressors and subsequently counsel these people about life changes that are often traumatic with long-term implications (Dziegielewski 2004). While as social workers we can account very well for our time and what we have done, we do not have objective, organised data indicating whether what we do makes a difference for the people we are serving.

This question about service outcomes is not unique to social work. Indeed, the impact of service has been the subject of discussions for the health professions over many years (Gibbons 2001). Professions that are more physically 'treatment based' as a result of a medical diagnosis appear to have access to a variety of standardised tools that will measure the patients' physical improvement and, by implication, the success of the clinician's intervention. For health professions working more broadly than in response to a medical diagnosis alone, some outcome measurement tools are available that focus on specific mental conditions and provide scores for pre- and post-interventions (Shapiro et al. 2009). However, for social workers in a wide variety of health clinical settings, client psycho-social concerns tend not to be defined by clear and exclusive diagnostic groupings (Auslander 2000).

For example, clients may be referred to social work because of domestic violence or expressed feelings of lack of control rather than a clear statement about a state of depression. Included in these people's range of concerns could be issues of relationship, finance, housing and employment. How do social workers assess the impact of their work with such a complex array of client concerns?

In the Hunter region of New South Wales (NSW), Australia, a group of social workers working in health, was interested in finding a way of asking clients to identify their concerns, in their own words, at the commencement of receiving social work services and then again after the work had concluded, with the aim of evaluating the impact or outcome on these clients' concerns. Our objective was to develop and test a tool that was more than a measure of satisfaction with social work services. Such measures often use survey questionnaires that provide simple feedback about the percentage of people satisfied with their service or session, people's level of engagement and if they would recommend the service to a friend. Satisfaction surveys do not really address underlying questions about clients' goal expectations and whether interacting with the social worker made a difference with regard to the issue/s being addressed (McNeil et al. 1998). The decision to undertake this task was also grounded in the contemporary demands for research-based evidence of practice effectiveness and research-based standards of excellence (Epstein 2001, p17). As Cheetham states:

> At this point in history, when good intentions, altruism and devotion to the disadvantaged are not accepted as sufficient justifications for Social Work's existence, its professional and public reputation and, most important of all, the standards of its services will be enhanced by good effectiveness research (Cheetham 1992, p265).

Our intention was to approach the problem from the standpoint of practice excellence, i.e. 'practice-based research' (Epstein 2001, p17). In other words, rather than seeking 'objective' measures of change that existed outside the client, we were interested in looking at the client's perception of goal attainment.

In launching out on a significant period of practice-based, practitioner-led research, the social workers were focusing on the principles and standards of their profession while addressing organisational and health context demands. Still, every effort was made to conduct all aspects of this pilot within sound, professional research standards (Australian Association of Social Workers 2003). These require social workers to ground their research in principles of human rights and social justice, to address client needs and organisational goals (Australian Association of Social Workers 2010). Core to this practice-based research (PBR) process is critical reflection on the application of social work knowledge, values and skills (Fook 2002). The challenge in this process was to develop rigour in research while privileging client experiences and rights.

Literature review: finding the path through the undergrowth

In 2005, Hunter New England Health (HNE) social workers were granted funding to employ a project worker for three months (May–August 2005) to conduct a literature review and search for social work service outcome-measurement tools under the guidance of a small steering committee. The literature search focused on the behavioural sciences databases available such as PsycInfo, Cumulative Index to Nursing and Allied Health Literature (CINAHL), PubMed and Newcastle University's Library Catalogue (NEWCAT). Initial searches concentrated on identifying studies on outcome measures for social work, evidence-based practice, measurement tools and questionnaires in use in social work settings. Searches were then widened into related disciplines such as psychology, occupational therapy and speech pathology. As articles were identified, their reference materials were cross-checked for other promising articles. In addition, internet searches were conducted to identify other measurement tools and the arrangements for their purchase or viewing.

Thirty tools that appeared relevant to social work were identified and reviewed by both the project's steering committee and a small group of senior clinicians. A short list of 11 tools was compiled including the Hospital Anxiety and Depression Scale (HADS) (Zigmond & Snaith 1983), Patient Generated Index (PGI) (Ruta & Garratt 1994), General Health Questionnaire (GHQ) (Goldberg & Hillier 1979) and Session Ratings Scale (SRS) (Duncan et al. 2003). These 11 tools were presented to a broad forum of social workers to determine each tool's appropriateness for their client groups, and for the ease of use by both clinicians and clients. The social workers came from a range of settings including acute, rehabilitation and mental health hospitals, community health generalist teams, sexual assault and child protection services, and adolescent and children's services. The feedback on the tools provided information about clinicians' views about utility and limitations of these tools. Existing psychology-based, questionnaire-type tools were considered too prescriptive in their questions and the quality of life tools too general for the purpose of evaluating social work outcomes. There was no clear winner from amongst those reviewed but six were considered as potentially useful in specific settings.

Ultimately clinicians preferred tools that allowed clients greater freedom to identify and assess their own issues. This finding echoed similar studies of social workers' approaches to outcomes tools (Felton 2005). A major stage one project recommendation was to commence the development and trial of a specific outcome tool for social work (Murphy 2005).

At the crossroads: follow the yellow brick road or blaze a new trail

The conclusion of stage one of the social work outcomes project saw the formation of a new steering committee to further develop the recommendations made at the end of the literature review process. This group consisted of the Director of Allied Health Services (HNE), Director of Social Work (Greater Newcastle Hospital Group), the project worker involved in stage one, a lecturer in social work from Newcastle University and a clinical coordinator from Mental Health Services.

The steering committee discussed the potential for creating a tool applicable in a broad range of social work health settings that could be the basis for *prospective* rather than *retrospective* clinical data mining (CDM) (Epstein & Joubert 2010, p322). The latter is the more typical and less labour-intensive path that most clinical data miners take.

Based on the social work consultation process, the following tool development principles were defined:

- free text space in which the client could define/describe their concerns
- measures both pre- and post-social work intervention
- be quick and simple to complete autonomously by the client.

The Patient Generated Index (PGI), a self-administered, quality of life tool originally completed by patients with lower back pain (Ruta & Garratt 1994), provided a model for an outcome tool development. This validated tool allows clients to describe an issue and then rate its importance relative to other issues. With permission from the author of the PGI, the tool was simplified with a view to its potential application in a wide variety of practice settings.

An eight-month period of steering committee meetings and consultation with social workers resulted in the development of the Client Outcomes Tool (COT). This process of development was aided by attendance at CDM workshops and consultations with Professor

Irwin Epstein from the Hunter College School of Social Work of the City University of New York.

Caution: steep incline ahead

Stage two of the project: trial of the COT

With further funding from the HNE Health Area Allied Health budget, a project worker was engaged for six months to trial and evaluate the COT between May and October 2006. As the previous project worker was not available to progress this work, a new project worker, familiar with the work to date, took on this next phase. Her responsibilities were to format the COT, put together an education package and conduct education sessions with social work centres in the properties of the tool, collate the data from the tools completed and provide basic analysis and recommendations.

Description of the COT

The COT (Appendix 1) has four main steps and two areas that provide free text for the client to write about issues and concerns impacting on their life. In the first step, clients are asked to name these concerns in their own words. They are not asked to rank these relative to each other using a weighting measure as in the PGI. In step 2, the pre-intervention measure utilises a 10-point Likert scale to measure the impact of each issue where 1 represents 'as bad as it can be' and 10 represents 'as good as it could be'.

The same 10-point Likert scale is used for step 3 where clients are asked to rate the issue after the social work intervention is completed (post-measure), and in step 4 clients are asked to rate the social work intervention as contributing to the resolution of the issue. The final section (step 5) is again one of free text asking clients to identify if there are other reasons contributing to the issues' resolution other than the social work sessions – i.e. those *ad hoc*, coincidental or confounder situations. For example, someone coming for financial counselling wins the lottery or the perpetrator of violence dies, leaving the client safe and without the need to establish safety plans. Clients were also asked to rank their general quality of life using the Likert scale.

Education of clinicians

The project worker conducted education sessions across 18 sites between June and September 2006. Social workers were also given detailed written instructions on specific criteria for when and how to introduce the tool to clients. These were:

- the client was over the age of 16 years
- pre-intervention questions were to be completed at either the beginning or end of the first contact
- in the acute settings, clients were to complete the post questions prior to discharge or when they had completed the social work intervention
- in a community setting, clients were to complete it at the end of the fourth counselling session if the sessions were continuing.

Social workers were requested to trial the tool over a three-month period with as many appropriate clients as possible. Social workers were also requested to critique the tool at the end of the trial period. Part of this critique was an examination of the concept of 'appropriate clients' for whom the COT could be administered.

Establishing the COT database

In total 108 completed COTs were returned from eight service sites by social workers predominantly located in city-based services and acute hospitals.

The data from each tool was entered in a Microsoft Access program and the results collated. Analysis of the client-defined issues began with open coding, which allowed for examination of the text so that categories and themes could be identified (Lofland et al. 2006).

These grouped, client-identified issues were then linked to National Allied Health definitions for Indicators for Intervention (IFI) as developed by the National Allied Health Classification Committee (NAHCC) (Australian Psychological Society Ltd 2008). The IFI categories are based on the International Classification of Function (ICF) dataset categories (World Health Organization 2001). The ICF dataset is an internationally recognised and validated classification system for coding a person's functioning rather than coding by medical diagnostic category. The ICF uses a bio-psycho-social model to help conceptualise and measure health-related issues on the basis of client reported information. Over 20 years the NAHCC in conjunction with the Australian Commonwealth Department of Health and Ageing undertook extensive research to develop a set of IFI for all allied health professions. Each IFI theme is based on a factor in a client's functioning or situation that requires allied health intervention. There are 37 IFI categories defined as social work indicators for intervention. The decision to link the HNE social work client-focused concerns to these nationally and internationally defined categories was an effort to relate the realities of social work practice to the larger organisational and global health service industry demands for rigorously researched outcomes of practice. The HNE COT project qualitative data was able to be linked to the following 12 IFI themes.

Table 2.1: Relevant IFI categories

IFI Theme	Theme descriptor
Emotional functions	Specific mental functions related to the feeling and affective component. Includes the appropriateness of emotion, regulation of emotion and range of emotion – sadness, happiness, love, fear, anger, hate, tension, anxiety, joy, sorrow, lability of emotion, flattening of affect.
Health services systems and policies	Services, systems and policies for preventing and treating health problems, providing medical rehabilitation and promoting a healthy lifestyle.
Family relationships	Including parent–child and child–parent relationships, siblings and extended family relationships.
Carrying out daily routine	Managing and completing the daily routine: managing one's own activity level.

IFI Theme	Theme descriptor
Economic self-sufficiency	Having command over economic resources from private or public sources in order to ensure economic security for present and future needs.
Intimate relationships	Includes romantic, spousal and sexual relationships.
Transport services, systems and policies	Services, systems and policies for enabling people or goods to move or be moved from one location to another.
Housing services systems and policies	Services systems and policies for the provision of shelters, dwellings or lodging for people.
Social security systems and policies	Services, systems and policies aimed at providing income support to people who, because of age, poverty, unemployment, health condition or disability, require public assistance that is funded either by general tax revenues or contributory schemes.
Legal services systems and policies	Services, systems and policies concerning the legislation and other law of a country.
Looking after one's health	Ensuring physical comfort, health and physical and mental wellbeing such as maintaining a balanced diet, an appropriate level of physical activity, avoiding harms to health, following safe sex practices, getting immunisations and regular physical examinations.
Sensation of pain	Sensation of unpleasant feeling indicating potential or actual damage to some body structure.

Mining the pilot project data: results

Figure 2.1 below depicts the percentage of client concerns linked to the 12 IFI definitions. The percentages for each category relate to the total of times the concern was mentioned whether it was listed as the first, second, third, fourth or fifth concern of the patient.

Figure 2.1: Client concerns by IFI category

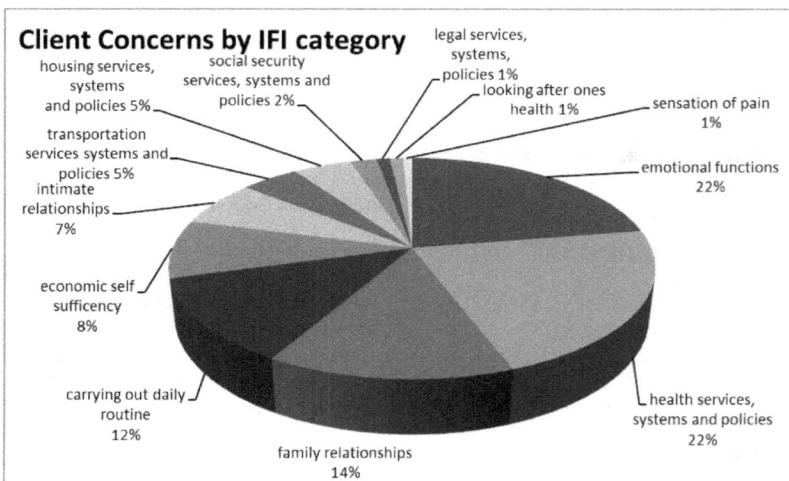

Client Concerns by IFI category

- legal services, systems, policies 1%
- looking after ones health 1%
- sensation of pain 1%
- emotional functions 22%
- health services, systems and policies 22%
- family relationships 14%
- carrying out daily routine 12%
- economic self sufficency 8%
- intimate relationships 7%
- transportation services systems and policies 5%
- housing services, systems and policies 5%
- social security services, systems and policies 2%

A closer examination of the top three areas of concern.

Emotional functions

Nearly one-quarter of the client concerns (22.5%) were about specific mental functions, which related to their feelings. This included the appropriateness, regulation and range of emotion, such as sadness, happiness, love, fear, anger, hate, tension, anxiety, joy, sorrow and lability of emotion. Some quotations included: 'Sad and worried about my husband's future', 'Worried that I will separate from my wife', 'I feel worthless', 'Anxiety, nervous problems', 'Depression', 'Panic attacks', 'My wife's death', 'Feeling sad and confused'.

Health services, systems and policies

Twenty-two percent of the client group were either confused or uninformed about the services that were available to them or the family member receiving treatment. They also expressed the need for social workers to explain treatment options in a non-medical way. For example:

> 'Where do I get home help from?', 'Needing to understand dialysis treatment in simple terms', 'Referral to community services', 'Help with managing my parents and the doctors', 'Nursing homes or hostels', 'Answers from medical staff that I can understand', and 'Information about hospital process'.

Family relationships

Fourteen percent of clients and their families sought assistance about dealing with the conflict they were experiencing with their parents, children, siblings and extended family members. Examples included: 'My ability to deal with family issues', 'Relationship with my kids', 'My ex-husband', and 'Extended family issues'.

Figure 2.2 demonstrates the change in the issue from the client's perspective. These results were achieved by measuring the difference between the Likert scale ratings pre- and post-social work intervention for the total group of first concerns, second concerns etc. regardless of what these concerns were about. The majority of clients only listed one concern. While for some clients the results indicate no change to the concerns post-social work intervention, the majority of clients indicate between one and nine points of positive change. The results that indicated a negative change, i.e. it would seem that the issue became worse after the social work intervention, were examined further. In some instances it appeared that the client misinterpreted the Likert scale because the comments in the final free text section described a helping relationship or positive experience of the social work intervention. This would not be expected if the issue had indeed become worse. These results were still included in the graph as this supposition could not be verified with the clients concerned and in reality for some clients' concerns could indeed become worse over the period of social work intervention.

Figure 2.2: Shift between pre- and post-intervention scores by concerns

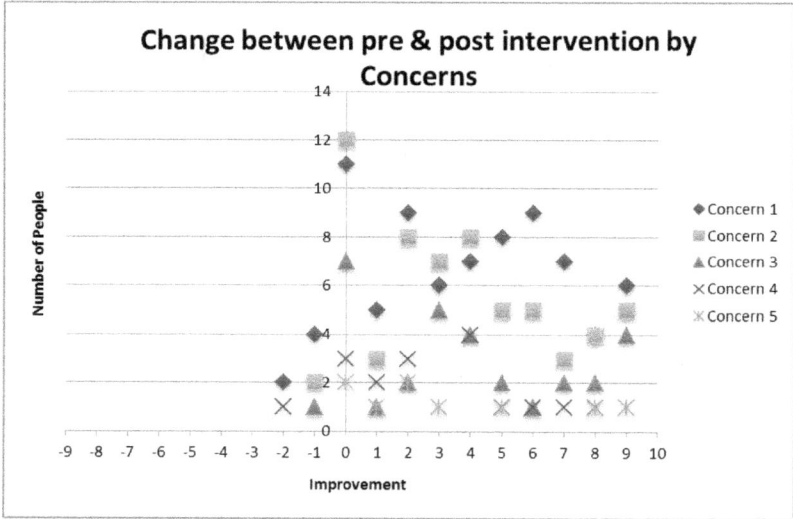

Figure 2.3 indicates that on average social work intervention was rated as being very helpful and contributing to the resolution of the issues, scoring 8.49 out of 10 for those who nominated one concern. Those with multiple concerns, up to five concerns, also rated the social work intervention very highly at 8.64 out of 10. These results compare favourably with earlier studies about patient and family satisfaction of social work services (Pascoe et al. 1983; McNeill et al. 1998).

Full details of the COT pilot results can be found in Montagnol, Hodgson, Giles and Rhodes (2008).

Figure 2.3: Client rating of social work support

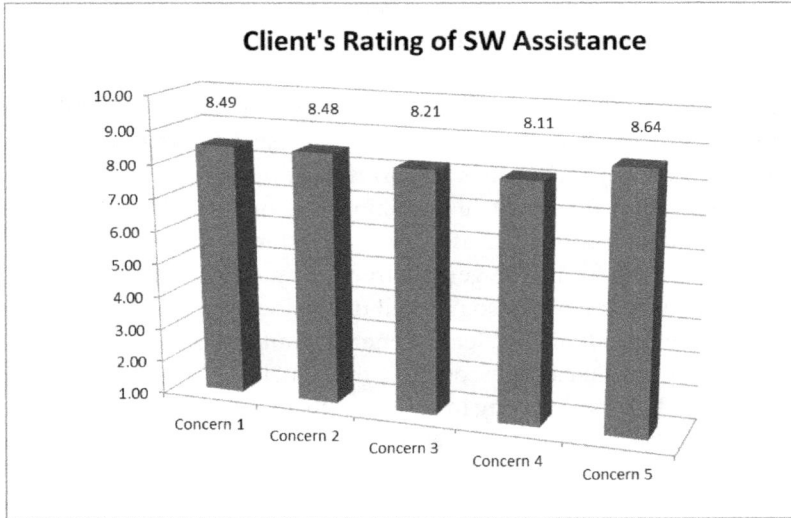

Client's Rating of SW Assistance

Concern 1: 8.49
Concern 2: 8.48
Concern 3: 8.21
Concern 4: 8.11
Concern 5: 8.64

Discussion

Client-perceived outcomes of social work services

The trial of the tool provided an extensive range of data for mining in relation to the outcomes of social work practice. Qualitative data was available in the free text of client concerns and quantitative data in the rating scales of feelings pre- and post-social work intervention as well as rating of the level of client support received from the social worker.

The results of the trial broadly indicate that:

a. social work interventions resulted in positive outcomes for clients in relation to their identified concerns

b. the level of support provided by social workers was predominantly rated as high.

Viability of an outcome tool

Overall the COT pilot feedback indicated general social worker agreement about the tool's usefulness in providing information on a client's experience of their contact with the social worker and as a means of genuine outcome measure. While this feedback indicates the viability of the COT, further refinement is required to enhance its application with a broad range of client groups and practice settings.

The general quality of life question was only completed by 57% of clients and was often missed in its position at the bottom of the first page of the form. The general free text question relating to other coincidental factors was also not well understood by clients who either did not complete it or used it as a general comments section to provide feedback about their sessions or about the clinician. No clients identified extraneous factors occurring in their lives that would otherwise account for the positive resolution of their issues. These pilot data may indicate these questions are superfluous to the tool's prime purpose.

Analysis of these data was also limited by the lack of a relative weighting for each of the client concerns against each other for importance. Hence, missing data precluded analysis of the relative importance of issues for clients; the first issue could be five times as important as the next issue but this was not known. These missing data could be valuable when considering questions of staff resources and length of time spent both with clients and in resulting indirect work.

Danger ahead: road subject to flooding

Facing the challenges of research in practice

Disappointingly only eight out of 18 trained sites (44%) returned completed tools. In reflecting on why this occurred it was noted that, while the tool was used by some hospital clinicians for single session interviews, it seemed to be most appropriate where there were several sessions over a few days or a week in the hospital or rehabilitation setting. The use of the COT in brief interventions with clients may require considerable change in the process of such sessions.

Some of the sites had severe staffing shortages, leaving no time for extraneous demands. Timing also contributed to the lack of response from those sites that did not receive training until later in the project period, leaving their completed tools outside the period for data analysis. Others stated they would have taken part with greater enthusiasm if routine departmental statistical data collection had ceased while the tool was being trialled. This response highlights the significance of clinical loads that are resourced without any allocation of time to participate in quality activities or research but a general expectation that these activities will somehow be included in a clinician's workload without an impact on direct client work.

In the generalist community health settings the issue of the period in which to have tools completed with clients was also highlighted. In this context the three-month pilot period was insufficient time to have completed interventions and ask the client to rank how this issue had resolved for them.

Some social workers also expressed concern that the outcome data had the unanticipated potential for use by managers for punitive evaluation of performance, particularly if clients ranked them poorly for support or resolution of their issue. This fear could cause social workers to selectively use it with clients who seemed to view social work intervention favourably thereby skewing the data. These concerns were acknowledged and some counter-balances were applied, e.g. the tool did not identify clinicians completing the tool. The tool recorded a client's medical record number (not name) as a way of matching the two halves of the form. At no point were further client details accessed to check which social worker was involved. While fear of negative consequences is acknowledged, all health employees are aware of and regularly participate in other performance review processes via medical record and other clinician intervention audits. Perhaps this response also relates to an acknowledged social work practitioner reluctance to participate in research (Hutson & Lichtger 2001, p154).

A major factor identified as promoting successful usage of the COT was strong and dedicated leadership at piloting sites. This leadership accounted for the majority of the tools being completed in the acute hospital system sites where the Director of Social Work was part of the steering committee and supervisor of the project worker. Other team leaders and site managers were strongly encouraged to participate as part of a quality improvement project activity. However, the challenges of trialling new practices and senior staff leave resulted in sporadic site-based leadership.

Applicability of the tool

In conjunction with consideration about which clients were appropriate to engage in responding to the tool was the question of when not to use the tool. Some areas identified by clinicians included those clients experiencing acute grief after the death of a relative or friend and those situations involving child protection concerns. In the latter a social worker's mandatory reporting obligation, considered to be in the best interest of the child, may be oppositional to the parents' current desires and hence be considered unhelpful and lacking in parental support. Social workers also debated the appropriateness of engaging with a carer to complete the COT if the patient was assessed as cognitively unable to participate in the process. In this circumstance it was deemed to be appropriate for the carer to complete the COT if that individual was the person with whom the social worker had the main contact.

From winding road to highway: a light up ahead?

In similar vein to many research projects, it seemed at this stage that developing the tool raised more questions than it provided answers. The project faltered between 2007 and 2008 due to insufficient funds for the employment of a consistent project worker and changes in membership of the steering committee. As a result the report remained in draft form until 2008 and unanswered questions and recommended changes to the tool remained untested. Without staffing consistency those remaining felt left in the wilderness.

However the Director of Allied Health and HNE Executive maintained an interest in outcomes of allied health services. Allied health interdisciplinary discussions resulted in occupational therapists, nutrition and dietetic staff, and speech pathologists expressing interest in adapting the COT for interdisciplinary use.

After sitting idly on the side of the road not really sure where to go next, it seemed like the main road was just over the next hill. With renewed enthusiasm, the COT was modified to incorporate feedback from the end of the second phase of the social work project and presented to the Allied Health Area Profession Directors in December 2008. Agreement was reached that an interdisciplinary COT was a worthwhile concept and further allied health funding should be allocated to a phase three trial of an allied health version.

Final reflections

COT development

On the basis of clinician feedback, the value of the free text components of the current tool is worthy of further consideration. Many clinicians reported that the clients had difficulty expressing their concerns in their own words, requiring considerable time spent in explaining the tool. The combined social work and allied health feedback indicates that one option may be to progress to a predetermined set of options.

A predefined list of concerns such as the well-researched IFIs would take less time to explain to clients and may seem less onerous to clinicians. However, such a decision takes the project back to the reason for its commencement, i.e. social workers were adamant that any outcome tool must be directly based in the local experiences of each client. In moving to a predetermined set of words, there is a risk that an individual client's meaning and experiences could be overlooked and the details of locally based health concerns unaddressed

Tool validation

In accord with measurement tool validation processes the COT development process has completed the stages of literature review, tool construction, initial piloting, adaptation and repeated piloting. Each of these stages seem to indicate that the COT can claim a basic level of face validity in that it reflects the real meaning of the concept under consideration, i.e. it reflects client-stated issues for practitioner intervention and client-driven opinion of the outcome of that intervention (Babbie 2004, pp143–45).

A more rigorous level of validation will be achieved as the tool is tested with larger numbers of clients and in specific settings. These future trials will provide further knowledge about the validity and the ability to generalise the COT.

Measuring the outcomes of social work and allied health practice

The context of health practice is fraught with severe funding constraints that threaten the viability of social worker and allied health positions resulting in internal competition for resources and power. In this context it is now essential that each professional group can clearly demonstrate value for money. It is no longer sufficient for social workers to simply rely on counting how many people are seen and what is done with those people. Such counting does not demonstrate either effectiveness or best practice. The creation of a tool that collects people's stated concerns and their direct feedback on the impact of social work and other allied health intervention is a genuine and valid attempt to keep indicators of outcomes grounded in ethical practice. Such practice commands respect for each client's experience of health and illness and a right to effective assistance with not only the physical factors influencing their health but also the psycho-social factors that strongly impact on wellbeing (Bywaters 2009).

The practitioner as researcher

Preliminary data from project phase three reflects the experience of the social work trial where, despite large numbers receiving training in the use and objectives of the COT, there was a relatively small allied health practitioner uptake. The same pressures of clinical workload and lack of resources were named as barriers to engagement in the trial. An additional barrier was the suitability of the COT for some of the professions. Once again this raises questions about the capacity of frontline clinicians to dedicate time to practice-based research (PBR) without major consideration of how to address direct client workload impact. While it is acknowledged there may never be enough funding for frontline clinical work, participation in practice research is vital to the understanding and improvement of that work and must be an essential practitioner activity.

The COT steering committee remain committed to the view that the tool has great potential as a practice tool, identifying client goals and providing guidance for clinicians in their follow-up work. This vision was challenged by the reluctance of some social workers and other allied health staff to work with the tool. Hutson and Lichtiger (2001) note the challenges for social workers in practice to step aside from their daily practice to engage with new approaches while Shapiro et al. (2009) identify the challenges for social workers to engage with and explore the concept of outcomes while also focusing on interventions and processes. Are these challenges underpinned by an inability to move beyond assessment to open communications about what really works in addressing client's needs and desires? Is there a reluctance to share conversations with clients about outcomes rather than being a directive and powerful health professional? Is this reluctance indicative of the hospital setting only? Are staff so busy completing the day-to-day tasks, covering absent colleagues, recording daily activity statistics, adjusting to working life, and incorporating home and work responsibilities, that there is no time or energy to think about the quality and appropriateness of their work? This could be an argument for *retrospective* rather than *prospective* CDM based on readily available data 'mined' only by motivated practitioner researchers.

Whatever the answers to these questions, as Rehr (2001) strongly proposes, reflective practice and practice research are both central to professional practice, to being accountable and to possessing full and complete information for decision-making. Both reflective practice and the research that follows engage practitioners in essential processes of correcting service systems and advancing the quality of care.

This project demonstrates that time, funding and maintaining vision and enthusiasm are important factors in achieving critically reflective practice and practice-based research. The five years of practice-based research (PBR) has been challenging. Sometimes the slow pace of change has been maddening, as has been the constant change of staff participating in the journey. In conducting practice-based research, do you ever arrive at your destination or does the road always lead somewhere else? At this point of the journey the project has achieved successful development of a valuable tool ready for targeted application and further growth of a dataset for mining. The process has engaged social work and allied health practitioners and managers in essential debate about outcomes in practice. The discussions and the data mining will continue even if the path gets a little overgrown in the meantime.

References

Auslander G (2000). Outcomes of social work intervention in health care settings. *Social Work in Health Care*, 31(2): 31–46.

Australian Association of Social Workers (2003). *Practice standards for social workers: achieving outcomes*. Canberra: AASW.

Australian Association of Social Workers (2010). *Code of ethics*. Canberra: AASW.

Babbie E (2004). *The practice of social research*. 10th edn. Belmont, California: Wadsworth/Thomson.

Bywaters P (2009). Tackling inequalities in health: a global challenge for social work. *British Journal of Social Work*, 39(2): 353–68.

Cheetham J (1992). Evaluating social work effectiveness. *Research in Social Work Practice*, 2(3): 265–87.

Duncan B, Miller S, Sparks J, Claud D, Reynolds L, Brown J & Johnson L (2003). The session rating scale: preliminary psychometric properties of a 'working' alliance measure. *Journal of Brief Therapy*, 3(1): 3–12.

Dziegielewski S (2004). *The changing face of health care social work: professional practice in managed behavioural health care*. 2nd edn. New York: Springer Publishing Company.

Epstein I (2002). Using available clinical information in practice-based research: mining for silver while dreaming of gold. *Social Work in Health Care*, 33(3–4): 15–32.

Epstein I & Joubert L (2010). Clinical data-mining in the age of evidence-based practice: recent exemplars and future challenges. In A Syvajarvi & J Stenvall (Eds). *Data mining in public and private sectors: organizational and government applications* (pp316–36). Hershey, New York: Information Science Reference.

Felton K (2005). Meaning-based quality of life measurement: a way forward in conceptualising and measuring client outcomes? *British Journal of Social Work*, 35: 221–36.

Fook J (2002). *Social work: critical theory and practice.* London: Sage.

Gibbons J (2001). Effective practice: social work's long history of concerns about outcomes. *Australian Social Work*, 54(3): 3–13.

Goldberg D & Hillier V (1979). A scaled version of the general health questionnaire. *Psychological Medicine*, 9(1): 139–45.

Hutson C & Lichtger E (2001). Mining clinical information in the utilization of social services: practitioners inform themselves. In I Epstein & S Blumenfield (Eds). *Clinical data-mining in practice based research* (pp153–62). New York: The Haworth Social Work Press.

Lofland J, Snow D, Anderson L & Lofland L (2006). *Analysing social settings: a guide to qualitative observations and analysis.* 4th edn. California: Thomson Wadsworth.

McNeil T, Nicholas D, Szechy K & Lach L (1998). Perceived outcomes of social work intervention: beyond consumer satisfaction. *Social Work in Health Care*, 26(3): 1–12.

Montagnol V, Hodgson F, Giles R & Rhodes D (2008). Social Work Outcomes Project final report, Pt 2. Hunter New England Health Service. [Online]. Available: www.hnehealth.nsw.gov.au/google_hneahs_search?cx=008965737287525525230% 3Am4ewdsvjeco&cof=FORID%3A11&q=%22Social+Work+Outcomes+Project% 22&sa=Go#163 [Accessed 25 March 2011].

Murphy G (2005). Social Work Outcomes Project final report, Pt 1. Hunter New England Health Service.

Pascoe G, Attkisson C & Roberts R (1983). Comparison of indirect and direct approaches to measuring patient satisfaction. *Evaluation and Program Planning*, 6: 359–71.

Rehr H (2001). Foreword. In I Epstein & S Blumenfield (Eds). *Clinical data-mining in practice-based research* (ppxv–xxiv). NY: Haworth Social Work Practice Press.

Ruta D & Garratt A (1994). A new approach to the measurement of quality of life: the patient generated index. *Medical Care*, 32(11): 1109–26.

Shapiro M, Setterland D, Warburton J, O'Connor I & Cumming S (2009). The outcomes research project: an exploration of customary practice in Australian health settings. *British Journal of Social Work*, 39(2): 318–34.

The Australian Psychological Society (2008). *Indicators for intervention (IFI) project*. Melbourne: Australian Psychological Society Ltd.

World Health Organization (2001). *International classification of functioning, disability and health (short version)*. Geneva: World Health Organization.

Zigmond A & Snaith R (1983). The hospital anxiety and depression scale. *Acta Psychiatrica Scandinavica*, 67(6): 361–70.

HNE Health Pilot Client Outcomes Tool : July to September 2006

Please complete this form to tell us about the areas you would like the social worker to help you with:

MRN: ....

DATE: ....

Tool Completed by
- Client ☐
- Family/Carer ☐
- Other ☐

Care Environment
- Community Health ☐
- Acute Hospital ☐
- Rehab ☐
- Mental Health ☐
- Sexual Assault ☐
- Other ☐
- Service Area ....

Gender
- Male ....
- Female ....

Age Group
- Under 20yrs ....
- 20's ....
- 30's ....
- 40's ....
- 50's ....
- 60's ....
- Over 70 yrs ....

Step 1 - Your concerns	Step 2 - Your Feelings (PRE)
In this section list in order of importance, up to five areas you would like the social worker to assist you with.	How have you been feeling about each of these issues in the last week? Circle a number between 1 and 10
	as Bad as could possibly be *as Good as could possibly be*
1. Most important concern	1 2 3 4 5 6 7 8 9 10
2. 2nd most important concern	1 2 3 4 5 6 7 8 9 10
3. 3rd most important concern	1 2 3 4 5 6 7 8 9 10
4. 4th most important concern	1 2 3 4 5 6 7 8 9 10
5. 5th most important concern	1 2 3 4 5 6 7 8 9 10
Compared to the issues listed above, how would you rate the other areas of your life.	1 2 3 4 5 6 7 8 9 10

July 7th 2006

81

HNE Health Client Outcomes Tool – Part 2

SERVICE COMPLETED: ....

SERVICE ONGOING: ....

Only complete this section when requested

Step 3 – Your Feelings This Time (POST)	Step 4 – Support	Step 5 – Significant Events
DATE: How have you been feeling about each of these issues in the last week? Circle a number between 1 and 10	On scale of 1–10, do you think the social worker made a difference to the issues you have sought support for?	Can you identify if anything else has happened in your life that may have affected the issues you have listed?
as *Bad* as could as *Good* as	*Little difference* *significant difference*	
1 2 3 4 5 6 7 8 9 10	1 2 3 4 5 6 7 8 9 10	....
1 2 3 4 5 6 7 8 9 10	1 2 3 4 5 6 7 8 9 10	....
1 2 3 4 5 6 7 8 9 10	1 2 3 4 5 6 7 8 9 10	....
1 2 3 4 5 6 7 8 9 10	1 2 3 4 5 6 7 8 9 10	....
1 2 3 4 5 6 7 8 9 10	1 2 3 4 5 6 7 8 9 10	....

Thank you for taking the time to complete this outcome tool. This will assist us in planning, delivering and improving social work practice

July 7th 2006

82

Chapter 3

Tackling solastalgia: improving pathways to care for farming families

Phoebe Begg and Sarah Thompson

The term 'solastalgia' (Albrecht et al. 2007) has been developed to describe the impact of drought on rural people. Challenging weather conditions, together with regulatory changes, uncertain markets and limited access to health services may contribute to high rates of mental health issues and suicide within Australian farm families.

The Farm Family Data Mining Project analysed electronic client data to report on the pattern and profile of farm family clients' uptake of health services in response to six discrete categories. The evidence gained in this research has challenged previous expectations about farming families and health service and informed changes in practice. The findings provide direction for future rural health policy development which improves responsiveness to the rural context and reflects the changing needs of farm families.

Key words: farm families, drought, data mining, community development, access, primary health care

In June 2005, following years of prolonged drought, the NSW Farmers Association invited key rural mental health stakeholders to a forum discussing how to best work together in addressing rural and remote mental health issues. A formal NSW Farmers Mental Health (NSW Farmers MH) Network was formed and a NSW Farmers Blueprint for

Maintaining the Mental Health and Wellbeing of the People on NSW Farms was developed (NSW Farmers Mental Health Network n.d.).

Within this macro context, on a micro level, in May 2006 the Rural Hunter Service Provider (RHSP) Network was established. The RHSP Network's aim was to coordinate and strengthen the local mental health system capacity and referral by linking to the rural financial counsellors, who have been identified as a first contact for rural people in crisis and the psychological/social support counselling services (Fuller & Broadbent 2006). A multi-sectored, multi-levelled and multi-method community action plan was developed. Rural community engagement should be multifaceted, occurring at multiple levels of the participation framework and ranges from engagement in rural policy development, through partnerships with agencies and consumers to plan and deliver local services, to individual engagement with programs (Kilpatrick 2009).

At the initial meeting of the RHSP Network a number of community service representatives expressed the position that farm families do not access health services. In contrast, health practitioner wisdom concluded that farm families did access health services. However, health service reports did not provide statistical data to support and quantify the claims of the health practitioners.

In order to quantify our practice wisdom, a smaller multi-disciplinary multi-levelled data-mining project team was established to harness Community Health Information Management Exchange (CHIME) data and report on farm family service uptake of Community Health Services. Community Health works with individuals, groups and other organisation to keep the community as healthy as possible. In this setting health workers take a holistic approach which encompasses physical, psychological and social wellbeing. This involves identifying health problems early, working with the community to promote health by changing influences outside the control of individual people and providing support, counselling or treatment for specific issues affecting health.

CHIME is an electronic client database which records all client contact and clinical notes. Clinical department specific service requests are recorded for each new episode of client contact. A new service request is generated when the episode of client contact has been closed for more than a three-month interval.

Literature review

Solastalgia is the pain or sickness caused by the loss or lack of solace and the sense of desolation connected to the present state of one's home environment. It is the homesickness you have when you are still at 'home' and the feeling you have when your sense of place is under attack. It is not just large-scale landscape changes such as loss of vegetation, dust storms, dead and starving animals. It is also smaller-scale events like the loss of the much loved farmhouse garden that finally trips people over into solastalgically induced depression and illness (Albrecht et al. 2007).

The impact of drought and solastalgia (Albrecht et al. 2007) are described as generalised distress and feelings of loss and bereavement which may lead to more serious health and medical problems such as drug abuse, physical illness and forms of mental illness. So powerful is the connection between a loved place and the experience of negative transformation that, for some people, suicide is seen as the only form of relief. This work seems to describe the underlying pain and distress experienced by Hunter farming families and resulted in the formation of both the NSW Farmers Mental Health (MH) and RHSP Networks.

In relation to health service uptake, the Australian literature suggests that farm families are historically perceived to only have a limited uptake of health services. The reasons for limited uptake include the stigma associated with acknowledging and seeking mental health information, alcohol misuse, social and geographic isolation and limited service options (Alston 2007). Alarmingly the literature also reports that deaths from suicide of male farmers and workers are approximately double that of the Australian male population (Page & Fragar 2002). The literature review also revealed a number of studies of drought response initiatives addressing the social and economic impacts of drought (Crocket et al. 2009; Tonna et al. 2009). Important in these is the process of social network analysis. The Fuller and colleagues' social network analysis (2007) involved a pilot survey of rural human service providers who work with mental health-related issues among farmers about their self-reported links between each other. The purpose was to inform improvements in this network and to serve as a baseline against which such improvements could be evaluated. This study, conducted under the auspice of FARMLINK, an Australian farming research organisation, in 'town C' concluded that the local service provider networks are not only about increasing or improving the referral process. The study found that increased links in information exchange and in working together are also important and indicate greater local mental health capacity-building and improved pathways to care.

The literature also suggests that multi-levelled rural community engagement in health should produce a system that recognises and responds to community needs in a way that is consistent with both community and health service norms and values. Community engagement will develop capacity of the community and health professionals and draw appropriately on community resources (Kilpatrick 2009).

While some of these findings may at first glance appear contradictory, practice wisdom suggests that farm families do support each other through tough times. Relationship challenges emerge post-drought when the emergency response is over and the financial situation has improved.

The literature review did reveal a gap in the research of studies which linked client characteristics, in particular gender, to service intervention, and correlated service network implementation and significant rainfall to service uptake. For the purposes of this study significant rainfall refers to rain in excess of 100 mm per month.

Methodology

This clinical data-mining project was undertaken by a multidisciplinary practitioner team. The project began with the development of a clear plan for analysis of existing client service access data. The aim was to link client service usage over time, with gender and service type and to correlate service usage with the formation of the two networks and rainfall patterns. The service delivery team were interested to know firstly, whether or not farming families were using the services provided and secondly, the timing of this service access. Finally, the team hoped to determine whether the patterns of service access altered with the formation of key social networks and according to improved climatic conditions of rain.

Consultation was undertaken with a number of groups. These groups included the CHIME team, the Hunter New England Health Human Research Ethics Committee and the Australian Centre for Agricultural Health and Safety Unit. The latter unit is a research centre within the Department of Public Health and Community Medicine at Sydney Medical School, University of Sydney, and situated in Moree, NSW. The aim of the centre is to assist rural Australians to attain improved levels of health and wellbeing by action to reduce the incidence and severity of injury and illness associated with life and work in agriculture (Australian Centre for Agriculture Health and Safety n.d.)

A project definition was developed of a farm client, to be someone who primarily lives on a farm and defines themself as a farmer. A coding process was also developed to identify farm clients registered on CHIME and involved typing the words 'farm client' on the third line of the address field. This uniform coding process ensured the reliability of the data. A list of existing CHIME data categories was identified to form the search variable for future CHIME reports. Age groupings were also established based on the life cycle.

Organisational context

This study is located in the Hunter and New England region, a rural Australian area of land approximately130,000 square kilometres with a population of 840,000 people. This area is located 240 kilometres north-west of Sydney, New South Wales, an eastern state of Australia. The area is dominated by farming communities, mines and wineries.

The study area contains three small townships, two larger regional centres, has three small hospitals, two multipurpose health centres and one Community Health team. Community Health provides multidisciplinary primary healthcare services to the hospitals and communities of the Muswellbrook and Upper Hunter Shires. At the time of this study, the disciplines of dietetics, social work, psychology, occupational therapy, speech pathology and nursing provided services to a farmer client base of approximately 1350 people residing in the three postcode areas of Muswellbrook, Scone and Merriwa (Australian Bureau of Statistics 2006a, 2006b, 2006c). There were no additional funded clinical Community Health positions created to provide services to farmers during the time of the study.

Sample

A snapshot of 158 farm family clients, accessing community and mental health services from 2002 to 2009, were identified by applying the data collection process described below. These farm clients were referred to a total of 404 community and mental health services.

Aims of the study

The initial project aims were to:

- track service provision to farm clients through service mapping to increase understanding of current service contact
- develop a baseline outcome measure to assess service initiatives
- identify the impact of the formation of the NSW Farmers Mental Health Network, the Rural Hunter Service Provider Network and major falls of drought-breaking rain
- target Upper Hunter Health Service planning as well as planning in partnership with the Rural Hunter Service Provider Network.

Data sources and collection process

All Community Health staff were asked to retrospectively code farm clients according to the above definition over the period from the introduction of CHIME in 2002 to 2006. Farm clients were then coded on an ongoing basis from 2006 to 2009. The coding process ensured that farm clients would appear in CHIME reports at the point of service contact, both retrospectively and prospectively.

A data request was then made to the CHIME team. Search variables included the client characteristic variables of gender and age distribution and the service intervention characteristics of date and type of service accessed.

A non-identifying Microsoft Excel spreadsheet was forwarded by the CHIME team for manual analysis. Client referrals were reported for each discipline and for the whole community health service.

Statistical consultation resulted in farm client referral data being broken into the following six discrete time categories:

1. baseline July 2002 to June 2005
2. establishment of the NSW Farmers Mental Health Network July 2005 to April 2006
3. launch of RHSP Network May 2006 to February 2007
4. major Rain 1 March 2007 to May 2007
5. major Rain 2 June 2007 to October 2007
6. major Rain 3 November 2007 to January 2009.

Farm client referral rates were then compared between five periods using a one-way ANOVA with post-hoc analysis using a Tukey test.

Results

The reported referral rates were significantly lower at baseline compared to all other periods. Figure 3.1 below plots referral numbers between July 2002 and January 2009. The mean +/−1 standard deviations for the first 20 data points were plotted. The referral rate was relatively stable from July 2002 until May 2005. After this time there is a significant increase, with the majority of data points falling above 1 standard deviations suggesting a shift in the mean.

The reported referral rates were significantly higher in 'major rain 1' than after the formation of the NSW Farmers Mental Health Network, after the formation of the RHSP Network and the implementation of the action plan and 'major rain 3'.

Figure 3.1: The number of farm clients accessing Community Health

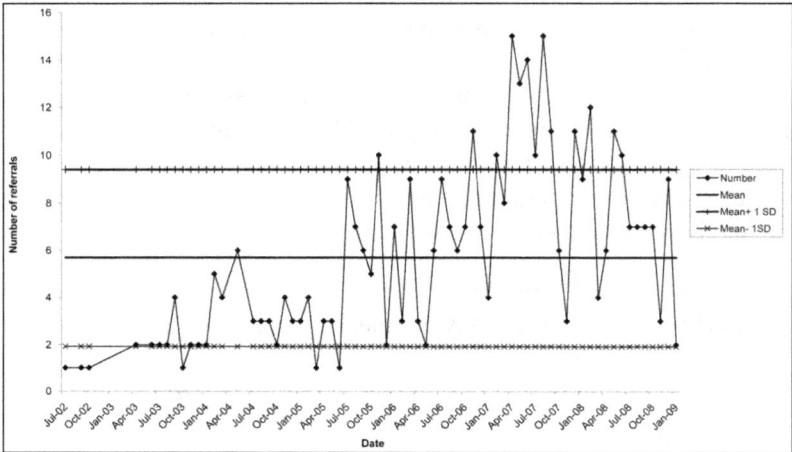

Figure 3.2 Referrals per service type July 2002–Jan 2009

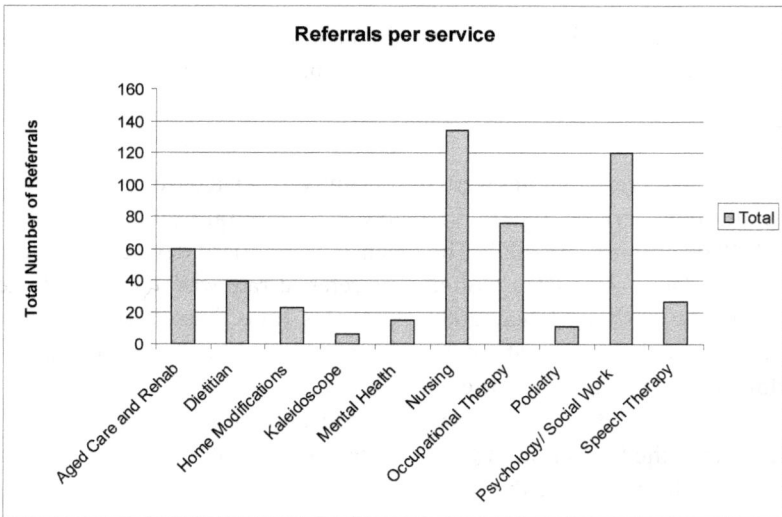

As seen in Figure 3.2 above, further analysis revealed that farm clients were accessing a broad range of service types and frequently accessing multiple community health services at any one time. The most frequently reported services accessed were psychology/social work, primarily for counselling; followed by community nursing, primarily for child and family health, dementia advice, foot-care, hearing, women's health, wound care and support and occupational therapy for independent living assessments, home modifications and children's clinics. This result aligns with the purposes of community health as outlined in the introduction.

Figure 3.3. The gender of farm clients accessing community health services from July 2002 to January 2009

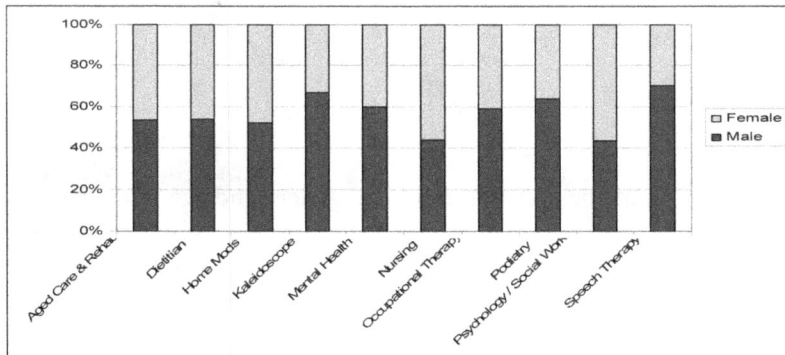

The data represented in Figure 3.3 above would suggest that community health services are accessible to both men and women. Nearly 50% of farm clients accessing community health services were male. This figure reduced to 43% for psychology/social work clients for early intervention/counselling in response to stress, adjustment, grief and loss, suicidality with no plans or intent, depression, parenting, self-harm, domestic violence, and other childhood behaviours. The figure increased to slightly more than 50% of farm clients accessing mental health services for suicidal plans with intent, schizoprenia, major depression and psychosis.

Figure 3.4. Age and gender of reported farm clients accessing community health services july 2002 to January 2009

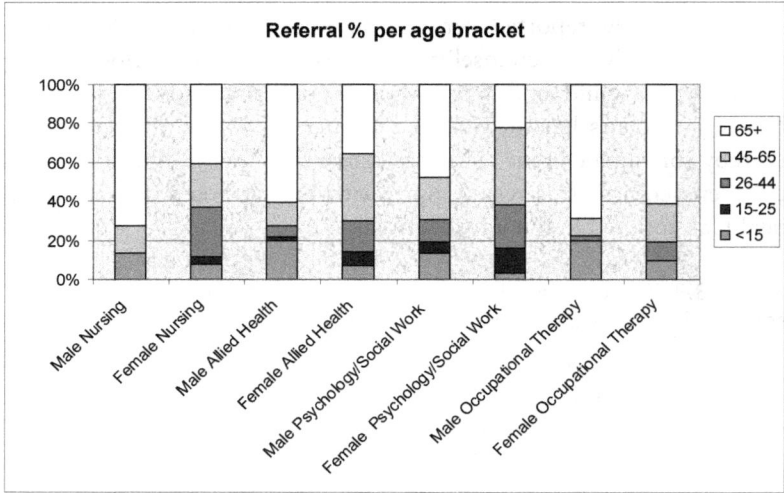

When farm client characteristics of gender and age were linked to service intervention, the complexity of rural generalist practice and distinct patterns of service usage emerged for nursing and allied health services as well as for the two most frequently identified allied health departments of psychology/social work and occupational therapy. Significantly, male farm clients over the age of 65 years and male farm clients under the age of 15 years access both nursing and allied health services more frequently than female farm clients of the same age bracket. Some of these services are likely to be for developmental issues not related to farming; for example, children attending speech pathology.

Discussion

The results of the farm family data-mining project suggest that increased numbers of farm family clients are being identified as accessing a broad range of community health services. The data also seems to confirm the literature in that network formations are strong influences in service usage, in this instance the formation of the NSW Farmers Mental Health Network in 2005 and the RHSP Network in 2006. A pattern of service usage has also emerged in relation to major rainfall events 1, 2 and 3. The reported referral rates were significantly higher in 'major rain 1' than after the formation of the NSW Farmers MH Network, after the formation of the RHSP Network and 'major rain 3'. The project team have concluded that the fact that farm clients are increasingly accessing a broad range of services would indicate that a multi-level and multi-disciplinary approach, consistent with best rural social work practice, is important when planning to increase client access for better mental health outcomes.

Data mining revealed that approximately 50% of the farm clients accessing community health services and 43% of farm clients accessing psychology/social work were male. These results are consistent with the service usage data of the New South Wales Rural Mental Health Support Line. Crocket, Hart and Grieg (2009) reported: 'The number of female and male callers was comparatively even. However, in any given month the numbers could be skewed significantly.' (Crocket et al. 2009, p282). Further analysis of CHIME gender breakdown reports suggests that male farm clients are accessing psychology/social work at a higher rate than the general community.

These findings are probably explained by the gender impacts of drought. Alston (n.d.) notes gender implications are seen to emerge as one of the most significant social impacts for farm family members. Farming women often manage multiple roles both on and off the farm. They juggle managing the farm office, with working off-farm to generate off-farm income and caring for the health and wellbeing of the family. The juggling of multiple roles often makes it difficult for women to attend appointments, particularly for early intervention services. For example, the data revealed that only three of the identified farm clients had accessed the women's health clinics. The women's health nurse has been practising in our area for approximately 20 years, providing a program of accessible clinics held in both the Upper Hunter health service centres as well as outreach facilities. Practice wisdom would have suggested that the women's health services would be an effective access point for other health service providers to access farm women. However, on this occasion the data has informed our practice and resulted in changes to the way health services are delivered. We now actively advocate for and educate farm women about the service and referral pathways to the women's health service.

In contrast to farming women, farming men become socially isolated and work longer hours on the farm to keep their stock alive. Male farmers witness the death of stock and loss of pastures on a daily basis, and consequently suffer an emotional impact. There is a strong link between the risk factor of social isolation and depression and this combined with the extra workload associated with drought may explain why there is a higher level of representation of male farm clients accessing mental health services.

This work is of significance as there is concern about men's mental health issues and use of services in Australia. Beyond Blue was established in October 2000 as a national five-year initiative to create a community response to depression, moving the focus of depression away from a mental health service issue to one which is acknowledged and addressed by the wider community (Beyond Blue n.d.a). The Beyond Blue website states:

> While rates of depression are not necessarily higher in rural areas compared to metropolitan areas, social isolation, lack of services and environmental factors – such as the current drought – may put some people at greater risk.

Beyond Blue also states that men are less likely than women to seek help for their health problems. Perhaps this is part of the male image of self-reliance: 'take charge', 'I can cope'. In addition, men are not very good at seeking out friends for support, or going to the doctor for professional help. When men do visit their general practitioner, they generally have short consultations, it's later in the course of the illness, and there is a tendency to not address significant health issues. All this means that men tend to be slow to acknowledge depression. Instead, they may be inclined to use unhelpful coping mechanisms such as increased drinking, working later and staying out rather than going home (Beyond Blue n.d.b).

Beyond Blue's claims are consistent with other mental health related research. Crosbie and Rosenberg (2007), reporting on Medicare funded mental health services, found:

- women aged 25–44 years were the greatest beneficiaries of the Medical Benefits Scheme (MBS) measures
- boys aged 5–14 years appear to be the only male group gaining access to MBS items more frequently than their female peers
- the uptake of new Medicare items relating to the use of social workers, occupational therapists and mental health nurses is negligible.

Likewise a study undertaken by Lifeline of the Lifeline 24 hour, 7 day per week telephone counselling service (Lifeline 2005) reveals that these services are twice as likely to be accessed by women. The highest number of calls to this service are from women aged between 35 and 44 years, with a higher proportion of female callers aged between 45 and 64 years in rural and remote areas. These results are similar to the community health farm client female profile. The Lifeline report also states that 'a high proportion of callers from rural/remote areas are married'.

A follow-up report by the Lifeline telephone counselling service (Lifeline 2007) revealed:

- 33.5% of callers were males
- the average age of both male and female callers was 45 years
- 45% of male callers lived alone while only 20% of male callers lived with their family
- the most frequent call time for rural and urban men is between 6 pm and 8 pm on a weekday, which is after business for most alternative counselling services
- the most frequent reasons provided by rural men for seeking telephone counselling through Lifeline were in relation to their mental health (18.1%), loneliness (11.9%), family and partner challenges (8.6%) and relationship breakdown and divorce (8.1%)

- of the mental health issues, the symptoms most frequently reported for rural men were depression (45%), anxiety (24%), mood swings (12%) and voices or hallucinations (11%)
- the most frequently reported triggers for rural men calling in relation to mental health issues were loneliness and insufficient support (47%) and general illness (17%).

These results are consistent with the data from the data-mining project which suggested that over 50% of farm clients accessing psychology/social work were recorded as never married, divorced or widowed, indicating a highly socially isolated client group.

Further analysis of the CHIME data referral resource report revealed that there were no recorded referrals made to psychology/social work by either the Drought Support Workers or the Rural Financial Counsellor. Although the project team report to have regularly linked farm clients to these services, cross-referral is not currently captured or available through CHIME reports. This may possibly explain why some of the RHSP Network partners expressed the view at the initial meeting that farmers did not access health services.

Limitations

This study was restricted to the Upper Hunter Community Health team, a public health service. The authors were not able to source data on farm clients accessing other health services such as a local doctor for their mental healthcare. Nor could the results be generalised across other rural communities and health services.

The project was reliant on busy clinicians and administration staff to code farm clients both retrospectively and on receipt of referral over a period of years. It was also reliant on the busy CHIME team to prioritise our data request, forward timely data results and clarify any areas of concern.

This busy project team did not have access to Statistical Package for the Social Sciences (SPSS) software. This created additional time demands, limitations in data analysis and reliance on external assistance.

The search variables were limited to existing CHIME data categories, and opportunities exist to add additional strength-based data categories at the next CHIME review. The current CHIME referral reports only reveal the referral source of total referrals made to a particular discipline-related department. Referral sources cannot be broken down on the basis of client age, gender, occupation or place of residence. Nor do the current report formats allow a clinician to track a client's entry into and pathway through the health service.

The results raised more questions than they answered, a finding common to data-mining research and other forms of research when they are done properly. The need to keep an open mind is always important in data mining or for any research (Epstein 2001). Further research is required to track farm clients' pathways into health and between the Community Health team.

Conclusions

This research prompted a significant shift from a 'discipline focus' on patterns of service delivery and uptake to an 'issue focus' through knowledge development in key areas, strengthening a team approach and documenting the outcomes of team work. This has promoted the transition of allied health professions from a position of being informed primarily by practice wisdom and generalised theory, to practice informed by their own evidence, reflection and theory testing (Posenelli et al. 2005).

The project results demonstrate the outcomes of multi-sector, multi-level and multi-method rural community engagement and working together to develop and deliver collaborative action plans to improve community linkages, promote information exchange, as well as hold mental health first-aid training and farm family gatherings.

An initial report of this study has gained organisational recognition and acknowledgement of the vital importance of the work of the Rural Hunter Service Providers Network. The work demonstrates that rural community health, i.e. accessible locality-based services, provides a unique range of early intervention services which complement the services provided by its network partners including the Medicare-funded mental health services and Lifeline telephone counselling service.

The identification of unique gender profiles of farm clients accessing community health services provides valuable practice-based evidence to develop understanding of the complexity of generalist rural practice and improve farm clients' pathways to healthcare. The identification of farm client contact across a range of health disciplines supports the imperative to provide targeted training in farm family cultural awareness, mental health literacy, mental health, building networks and maintaining cross-discipline and interagency relationships.

The provision of additional training to the clinicians identified as the most frequent primary contacts, namely nursing, social work and occupational therapy, is now recommended to ensure raised awareness of the unique and compound effects of drought on clients and their families' health outcomes, and thereby ensure appropriate effective care and referral pathways for farm clients. The complex client profile of the psychology/social work services adds to the ongoing calls for rural training and skill development to achieve timely, appropriate, effective and responsive healthcare with a focus on early intervention.

The evidence-informed practice has the potential to shape rural policy development which is responsive to rural context and reflects the changing needs of farm families. Consistent with the collaborative nature of the project, the project findings are regularly reported back to the Health Service, the NSW Farmers Mental Health Network, the Centre for Rural and Remote Mental Health and the Rural Hunter Service Providers Network to improve targeted service planning and performance monitoring. One example of effective use of the data is the implementation of collaborative initiatives between community health services, the Rural Division of General Practice and the drought support workers to increase female farm clients' uptake of women's health services. The frequent representation of younger males, particularly under the age of 15 years, accessing Community Health Service, provides a link to farm families and further opportunities for collaborative primary prevention. In this manner the farming families project findings have added to the body of knowledge related to farm clients' access to health services and statistically demonstrated improved pathways to community healthcare.

References

Albrecht G, Sartore G, Connor L, Higginbotham N, Freeman S, Kelly B, Stain H, Tonna A & Pollard G (2007). Solastalgia: the distress caused by environmental change. *Australian Psychiatry 7*, 15(s1): S95–S98.

Alston M (2007). Globalisation, rural restructuring and health service delivery in Australia: policy failure and the role of social work? *Health and Social Care in Community*, 15(3): 195–202.

Alston M (n.d.). Drought: a gendered experience. Centre for Rural Social Research. [Online]. Available: adl.brs.gov.au/data/warehouse/brsShop/data/alston23apr.pdf [Accessed 25 August 2010].

Australian Bureau of Statistics (2006a). *Basic community profile for postcode 2329. Table B42, Industry of employment by age by sex, 2006 Census of Population and Housing.* Canberra: Australian Bureau of Statistics.

Australian Bureau of Statistics (2006b). *Basic community profile for postcode 2333. Table B42, Industry of employment by age by sex, 2006 Census of Population and Housing.* Canberra: Australian Bureau of Statistics.

Australian Bureau of Statistics (2006c). *Basic community profile for postcode 2337. Table B42, Industry of employment by age by sex, 2006 Census of Population and Housing.* Canberra: Australian Bureau of Statistics.

Australian Centre for Agriculture Health and Safety (n.d.a). [Online]. Available: www.aghealth.org.au [Accessed 3 March 2011].

Beyond Blue (n.d.a) Our history. Beyond Blue: The National Depression Initiative [Online]. Available: www.beyondblue.org.au/index.aspx?link_id=2.22 [Accessed 28 April 2011].

Beyond Blue (n.d.). Depression in rural people. Beyond Blue: The National Depression Initiative [Online]. Available: www.beyondblue.org.au/index.aspx?link_id=84 [Accessed 28 April 2011].

Crocket JA, Hart L & Greig J (2009). Assessment of the efficacy and performance of the New South Wales Rural Mental Health Support Line. *Australian Journal of Rural Health*, 17: 282–83.

Crosbie D & Rosenberg S (2007). Mental health and the new Medicare services: an analysis of the first six months. COAG Mental Health Reform, Mental Health Council of Australia. [Online]. Available: www.mhca.org.au/.../AttachmentA-MHCAMedicareReportFirstSixMonths- Final.pdf [Accessed 28 April 2011].

Epstein I (2002). Using available clinical information in practice-based research: mining for silver while dreaming of gold. *Social Work in Health Care*, 33(3–4): 15–32.

Fuller J & Broadbent J (2006). Mental health referral role of rural financial counsellors. *Australian Journal of Rural Health*, 14(2): 79–85.

Fuller J, Kelly B, Sartore G, Fragar L, Tonner A & Pollard G (2007). Use of social network analysis to describe service links for farmers' mental health. *The Journal of Rural Health*, 15(2): 99–106.

Kilpatrick S (2009). Multi-level rural community engagement in health. *Australian Journal of Rural Health*, 17: 39–44.

Lifeline (2007) Help-seeking behaviours in rural men (Lifeline calls) Lifeline profile 4 September 2007. [Online]. Available: www.lifeline.org.au/About-Lifeline/Publications-Library/Lifeline-Publications/default.aspx [Accessed 28 April 2011].

Lifeline (2005). Profile of rural and metropolitan telephone counselling service users (Lifeline calls), Lifeline profile. [Online]. Available: www.lifeline.org.au/ArticleDocuments/124/lifeline_calls_profile_no_2.pdf.aspx [Accessed 28 April 2011].

NSW Farmers Mental Health Network (n.d.). [Online]. Available: www.aghealth.org.au/blueprint/ [Accessed 3 March 2011].

Page A & Frager LJ (2002). Suicide in Australian farming, 1988–1997. *Australian and New Zealand Journal of Psychiatry*, 36: 81–85.

Posenelli S, Joubert L, Power R, Vale S & Lewis A (2005). Managerial collaboration through allied health data-mining: the St Vincent's health experience. *Journal of Social Work Research and Evaluation*, 6(2):167–175.

Tonna A, Kelly B, Crocket J, Grieg J, Buss R, Roberts R & Wright M (2009). Improving the mental health of drought-affected communities: an Australian model. *Rural Society*, 19(277–370): 296–305.

Chapter 4

Mending bones and maximising independence: data mining an orthopaedic rehabilitation inpatient independent living unit

Jenny Swancott

'If you keep on doing what you've always done, you'll keep on getting what you've always got'. W Bateman

This was the scenario on our orthopaedic rehabilitation ward independent living unit (ILU) which commenced in the mid 1990s. Since that time the ILU staff had not systematically reviewed its utilisation and/or its outcomes. The staff simply assumed that the ILU was a useful resource assisting with assessments and discharge planning for patients. But was this the case? What was the impact of ILU trials? Could we possibly improve on our ILU clinical practice? If so, how?

Utilising clinical data mining (CDM) (Epstein 2010) as an evaluation methodology, the ensuing self-study indicated that an ILU trial was helpful in identifying those patients who could be safely discharged back to living in the community. It demonstrated that age, cognition and type of injury influenced ILU trial outcomes. New learning resulted regarding staff assumptions of a 'home-like nature' in the ILU and about patients and carers as active partners in the rehabilitation and decision-making processes. From the patient perspective the review revealed how relocation to the ILU could be stressful. It also highlighted the importance of a person-centred multidisciplinary approach in which the staff–patient–carer partnership is vital to maximising independence.

Key words: independent living unit, discharge planning, orthopaedic rehabilitation

Simply described, the ILU is a large single room in an orthopaedic rehabilitation ward with a patient bed, ensuite, a table and chairs, sink and bench space with a microwave for small meal preparation, tea and coffee making facilities, refrigerator, and space for a carer's bed. It is located near the activities of daily living (ADL) kitchen where ILU patients can also prepare meals using the oven or grill. An ILU trial assists in making assessments for selected patients prior to discharge to their own home or other accommodation.

The multidisciplinary team providing ILU patient services commenced a collaborative and systematic CDM analysis of the types of patients referred to the ILU, the reasons for referral and the outcomes of trial periods. Further, the team wanted to know if an ILU trial was helpful in discharge planning for health staff, patients and carers. The team also wished to consider how ILU documentation could be improved for future study and decision-making.

In effect, this study provided an opportunity for the team to collaboratively participate in a quality improvement activity relevant to each member's clinical practice. Like other practitioners before them, they were aware that this kind of a reflective data gathering and analysis process could be an experience with the potential to enhance effective multidisciplinary team relationships (Hutson & Lichtiger 2001; Posenelli et al. 2005).

A multidisciplinary project group of three social workers, an occupational therapist, a dietician and a nurse formed the project team. An audit proforma was developed with input from all staff. Due to work commitments and staff rotations the project team became the three social workers and an occupational therapist. Starting with a brief review of the literature, the team were surprised not to find articles about hospital ILUs. Knowing this, the team members were further motivated to write about the process and results of the self-study. The project team consulted twice with Professor Irwin Epstein about data-mining methodology, and the HNE Division of Allied Health provided funding to assist in the data collection process. Project approval was gained from the NSW Human Research Ethics Committee, Hunter New England Area Health Service.

Literature review

Discharge planning is regarded as a complex activity involving multi-disciplinary assessments, education and training of patients and carers, and collaborative work with patients and carers to develop planned treatment and discharge goals (Meier & Purtilo 1994, p365; Haas 2005). Patients requiring especially sensitive and responsive discharge planning include those who have complex care needs, a physical disability, cognitive impairment (for example, dementia), are old, or who have a carer (NSW Health 2007, pp7–11). In discharge planning, the patient's social context requires careful consideration, particularly for frail, older patients and those with an elderly carer (Manthorpe 2009).

Families are recognised as playing a key role in supporting patients when they return home from hospital, particularly with regard to frail older patients (Bauer et al. 2009). Accordingly patients and carers are central to treatment and discharge planning decision-making (Glazier et al. 2004; Petersson et al. 2009).

Whenever possible, patient involvement in goal setting is regarded as best practice (Sivaraman Nair 2003; Glazier et al. 2004). This involvement increases patient motivation in the identification and maintenance of personally meaningful healthcare goals (Barclay 2002; Sivaraman Nair 2003; Glazier et al. 2004; Christianson 2005). Collaborative and relevant short or long-term goals are best expressed in functional, non-technical language as realistic and measurable objectives (Becker et al. 1974; Barclay 2002; Black et al. 2010). In a rehabilitation context these frequently include patient ability to perform activities of daily living (ADLs) such as personal care, toileting, mobility, meal preparation and medication management (Christianson 2005).

While the benefits of collaborative partnerships with patients and carers are clear, there are also constraints in this process. These constraints include the influence of the institutional environment (Efraimsson et al. 2006; Moats 2006); differing staff, patient and carer expectations regarding the impact of illness, injury and impairment (Purtilo & Meier 1993; Sivaraman Nair 2003; Glazier et al. 2004); and differing interpretations of 'independence' (Barclay 2002). Underpinning these differences are the world views, backgrounds, experiences and value differences which health staff, patients and carers bring to conversations relating to treatment, rehabilitation and goal setting, including issues of institutionalisation and learned helplessness (Haas 2005).

Assessments associated with discharge planning generally occur in structured ward environments. Despite there being a multitude of articles discussing hospital discharge planning (see, for example, McMurray et al. 2007; Popejoy et al. 2009), as indicated earlier an extensive literature review did not locate any articles discussing discharge planning and an ILU trial in hospital.

In the absence of published research, clinical data mining was considered to be a highly appropriate methodology for studying an ILU on a government-funded hospital orthopaedic rehabilitation ward. As Epstein states: 'at their least elaborate and most descriptive, CDM studies produce invaluable information about client profiles, services received, and outcomes achieved' (Epstein 2010, p13). However, the 'ultimate purpose (of CDM) is to enhance clinical awareness and to improve clinical and programmatic decision-making based on a reflective process of research enquiry' (Epstein 2010, p22).

Organisational context

The Royal Newcastle Centre (RNC) is an 84-bed health facility located 150 kilometres north of Sydney, NSW, Australia. Treatment specialities include orthopaedics, orthopaedic rehabilitation, rheumatology, urology, ophthalmology, diabetes, dermatology, immunology and podiatry. The orthopaedic rehabilitation ward has had an ILU since the mid 1990s. The multidisciplinary team are highly committed to the value of this unit such that when the Royal Newcastle Centre (RNC) was relocated to another site in April 2006 the ILU was regarded as an essential component of the new rehabilitation centre design.

Methodology

Using CDM methodology the files for 22 patients admitted between April 2006 and April 2009 were queried to extract data about:

1. demographics of patients undergoing an ILU trial (including reason for admission to hospital, family and community services supports)
2. reasons for ILU trials
3. processes central to ILU trials including admission, assessment and ILU discharge
4. trial outcomes for patients, carers, and staff, including discharge destination
5. adequacy of documentation.

Sample

A list was generated of all patients admitted to the orthopaedic rehabilitation ward between April 2006 and April 2009 who had then been accommodated in the ILU room during their stay on the ward. As the ILU room is part of the bed stock on the ward, and ILU trials are planned to be for two nights or more, those patients whose length of stay (LOS) in the ILU was less than two nights were not regarded as having been accommodated in the ILU for the purpose of a trial. These patients were removed from the study sample.

The files of the remaining patients were reviewed to determine if they had completed an ILU trial. Twenty-two patients were identified as having undertaken a trial in the study period. These files were reviewed and a Microsoft Excel spreadsheet created. A thematic analysis was conducted of the documented processes associated with ILU trials; that is, staff discussions with the patients and carers concerning reasons for recommending a trial, the period leading into the trial, the trial period itself, patient and carer responses to the trial and its outcomes.

Aims of the study

The aims of this CDM project were:

1. identify reasons for an ILU trial referral
2. identify outcomes of ILU trials
3. develop ILU trial practice principles
4. improve ILU documentation.

Results

Patient demographics

Table 4.1 indicates 13 patients (59.1%) were female and nine male (40.9%). Only five (22.7%) had a carer involved. These carers comprised two husbands, a wife, a daughter and a daughter-in-law. Nineteen patients (86.4%) were born in Australia. The remainder were born in England, India and Poland.

Average patient age was 72.7 years, ranging from 29 to 99 years. Reflective of this wide variation, the standard deviation for age was 20.04 years. Fifteen patients (68.2%) were aged over 70 years. Nine patients (40.9%) were widowed. Six patients (27.3%) were married or in de facto relationships, four (18.2%) were separated, two (9.1%) were single and one (4.5%) was divorced.

Twenty patients (90.9%) lived in urban areas. Nineteen (86.4%) lived in a home or unit. Two (9.1%) lived in a caravan and one (4.5%) rented a shed. Fifteen (68.2%) owned their home or unit, four (18.2%) rented privately, and two (9.1%) lived in public housing. One patient (4.5%) lived in a relative's home.

Fourteen patients (63.6%) lived alone. Three (13.6%) lived with their spouse or partner, two (9.1%) lived with their spouse or partner and one of their adult children, two (9.1%) lived with one of their children and one (4.5%) lived with their dependent child.

Fifteen patients (68.2%) were retired from the labour force. Three (13.6%) were employed. One (4.5%) was unemployed and seeking work. One (4.5%) was of working age and receiving a government parenting payment, another received a disability support payment, while another worked part time and received a government payment.

Twenty patients (90.9%) were classified as public or non-chargeable patients, that is, their hospital care was paid for by the government. Two patients (9.1%) injured in car accidents were eligible for the NSW Motor Accident Authority Third Party and Lifetime Care and Support Schemes. Both these schemes cover hospital costs of eligible patients. Although all the patients were eligible for government-funded health benefits, their widely varying demographic profiles alone illustrate the challenge that discharge planning represents for this patient population.

Reasons for admission to hospital

Twelve patients (54.5%) required orthopaedic admission for injuries associated with a fall. Motor vehicle accidents resulted in three (13.6%) admissions and three patients (13.6%) were admitted following non-traumatic spinal cord injury. One patient (4.5%) was admitted with an infection post-elective surgery, two patients (9.1%) were admitted due to pain and one (4.5%) for pressure area management.

Table 4.1: Patient demographic matrix

Patient * = has carer	Female	Born in Australia	20-29	30-39	40-49	50-59	60-69	70-79	80-89	90+	Lives alone	Own home	Retired	Public Patient	Fall	MMSE completed	Family assistance	Community Services
1	X	X							X		X	X	X	X	X		X	X
2	X	X							X		X		X	X	X		X	X
3		X	X											X				
4*	X	X							X			X	X	X	X	X		
5		X							X		X	X	X	X	X	X	X	
6		X					X				X	X		X	X	X		X
7								X			X	X	X	X			X	
8	X	X								X	X	X	X	X	X		X	X
9*	X	X								X		X	X	X	X	X		
10*		X					X					X	X	X		X	X	X
11*	X	X						X				X	X	X	X	X	X	X

Patient * = has carer	Female	Born in Australia	20-29	30-39	40-49	50-59	60-69	70-79	80-89	90+	Lives alone	Own home	Retired	Public Patient	Fall	MMSE completed	Family assistance	Community Services
12*	X	X							X		X	X	X	X	X	X	X	X
13	X								X		X	X	X	X	X	X	X	X
14	X									X	X	X	X	X	X	X	X	
15		X				X					X					X		
16	X	X								X	X	X	X	X		X	X	X
17		X							X			X	X	X	X	X		
18	X	X							X		X	X	X	X	X	X	X	X
19	X	X	X											X				
20		X			X						X					X		
21		X		X							X					X		X
22	X	X			X						X	X						
%	59.05	86.36	45.45	45.45	13.63	0	9.09	13.63	40.90	13.63	63.63	68.18	68.18	90.90	54.54	54.54	68.18	50

Family support and community services accessed pre-admission

Table 4.2 outlines family and community service supports pre-admission and on discharge. Five patients (22.7%) received no assistance from either family members or community services prior to admission. With the exception of one patient, all five were less than 50 years of age. Six patients (27.3%) who received assistance from family members, and nine (40.9%) who received assistance from family and community services were aged over 70, while the two patients (9.1%) who received assistance only from community services were aged between 30–39 and 60–69 years of age respectively.

Table 4.2: Family and community service supports

Type of support or service	Family support		Community services	
	Pre-admission	Discharge	Pre-admission	Discharge
Grocery shopping	10 (45.5%)	12 (54.5%)	3 (13.6%)	4 (18.2%)
House cleaning	7 (31.8%)	8 (36.4%)	8 (36.4%)	9 (40.9%)
Meals	9 (40.9%)	12 (54.5%)	1 (4.5%)	0 (0%)
Transport	8 (36.4%)	13 (59.1%)	1(4.5%)	10 (45.5%)
Laundry	8 (36.4%)	8 (36.4%)	1 (4.5%)	3 (13.4%)
Finances	8 (36.4%)	9 (40.9%)	0 (0%)	0 (0%)
Medication management	3(13.4%)	3(13.4%)	1 (4.5%)	3 (13.4%)
Personal Care	3 (13.4%)	4 (18.2%)	2 (9.1%)	8 (36.4%)
Commode emptying	0 (0%)	1 (4.5%)	0 (0%)	1 (4.5%)
Pet care	0 (0%)	1 (4.5%)	0 (0%)	0 (0%)
Co-resident carer	5 (22.7%)	6 (27.3%)	NA	NA
Nursing	NA	NA	4 (18.2%)	7 (31.8%)
Package of care	NA	NA	0 (0%)	7 (31.8%)
In home respite	NA	NA	0 (0%)	1 (4.5%)
Residential aged care respite	NA	NA	0 (0%)	1 (4.5%)
Spinal Cord Injury Service	NA	NA	0 (0%)	2 (9.1%)

ILU Admission

All ILU trials were initiated by health staff concerned about the patient's or carer's capacity to successfully manage on return home. These concerns resulted in three patients (13.6%) who demonstrated a lack of initiation of ADLs while on the ward and five patients (22.7%) identified as not managing well pre-admission to hospital. Eight patients (36.4%) had a decrease or a negative change in mobility. One of the five carers indicated a need to know what level of care their relative required. An ILU trial was recommended for the four other patients (18.2%) with carers to assess the carers' ability to manage following increased patient care needs. The remaining patient was referred following an extended hospital stay and concern about ADL management within a limited time frame.

A Mini Mental Status Examination (MMSE) was conducted by the medical team for twelve (54.5%) patients as a standard component of their assessment. These patients ranged from 61–99 years of age with the average age of the patients being 82 years. A score of 25 or more signifies normal cognition (Hecker 2002; Gazewood 2009). Ten (83.3%) patients scored less than 25, including four of the five patients who had a carer. Nine (75%) of these 12 patients had fallen, resulting in a fractured femur. One patient, and another not in the MMSE cohort, also had cognitive assessments associated with legal and discharge decision-making, and had difficulty understanding the need for an ILU trial.

As Figure 4.1 indicates, prior to admission, 12 patients (54.5%) mobilised independently without aids and one patient (4.5%) mobilised independently in a manual wheelchair. Five patients (22.7%) mobilised using a walking stick and four patients (18.2%) mobilised with a frame. At the time of the ILU trial, two people (9.1%) used walking sticks, two (9.1%) Canadian crutches, twelve (54.5%) small frames, two people (9.1%) a Forearm Support Frame (FASF) and four (18.2%) a wheelchair.

Fourteen of the ILU trials (63.6%) occurred between Monday and Friday, with eight trials (36.4%) occurring over or incorporating a weekend. Trials lasted an average of three days and two nights.

Figure 4.1: Mobility pre-admission, during ILU trial and at discharge

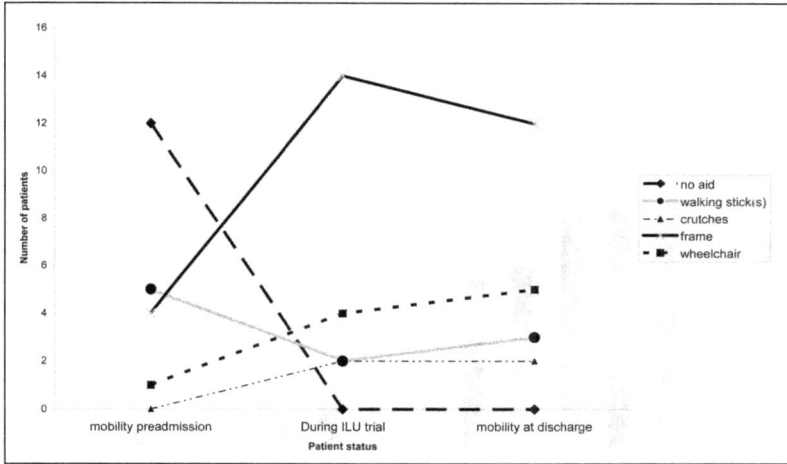

Activities of daily living during ILU trials

Patient or carer capacity to initiate and safely complete ADLs was a key determinant regarding appropriateness of patient discharge to community living. In particular, patients and carers were assessed for safe mobility and independence. For example, the ability to get in and out of bed, transfer on and off a chair or wheelchair and the toilet, prepare a meal and house cleaning. The selection of assessable activities was related to those which the patient or carer had not demonstrated on the ward and completion of which was essential to returning home safely.

An individualised program was developed for each patient (Meier & Purtilo 1994). Figure 4.2 indicates the range and frequency for each of these assessed ADLs during the trial period. There were a number of common ADLs, with five patients (22.7%) having unique activities. These included a parent caring for their child overnight while in the ILU and another patient being able to complete their activities of daily living within the periods available when not on bed rest. One patient needed to manage a urinary catheter, another needed to independently don and doff an ankle foot orthosis, a device that supported his weakened leg and enabled him to mobilise safely and independently, and a carer was responsible to maintain his wife's skin integrity.

Figure 4.2. Activities of daily living in ILU

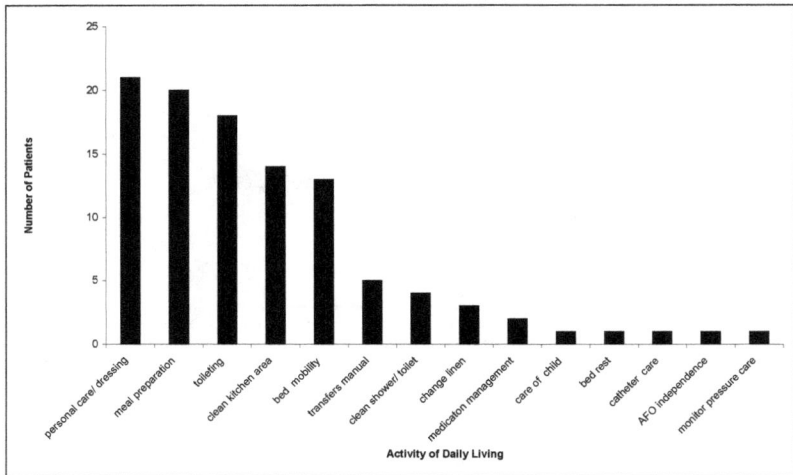

Outcomes of ILU trials

The ILU trials assisted health staff to assess patient/carer capacity to initiate ADLs, their safety when performing these activities, and the activities for which they required assistance or supervision. For example, the occupational therapist was better able to determine John's[1] equipment needs.

The ILU trial also helped patients and carers in their decision-making regarding their discharge care needs. Jane's family recognised her need to have a full-time companion in order to return home safely. A trial helped with determining the appropriate discharge destination for Sharon, the oldest patient, whose family believed she needed hostel care. Sharon, who lived alone, demonstrated management of night-time care and reheating of frozen meals. With assistance for personal

---

1 Names have been changed to ensure confidentiality.

care, Meals on Wheels and family support, Sharon returned home. Gail, on the other hand, chose to go to a low-care residential facility despite managing in the ILU.

Patients had rehearsal opportunities familiarising themselves with prior and new activities necessitated by their medical conditions. With the exception of Jane, the other patients demonstrated a willingness to initiate ADLs themselves. Anne, who had lost confidence in her ability to manage at home, reported she felt more able to cope at home following the trial. A community health service provider, who had accepted Anne's referral following a recent prior hospital discharge, did not accept Anne's re-referral as she was too highly functioning. Gary and Ian both had significant cognitive impairment, but capacity to make their own decisions made possible initiation of ADLs, and returned to their previous accommodation.

Cathy, sole carer of her school-age child, and now mobilising in a wheelchair, was able to care for her child in the ILU. Brian, an older spinal cord injury patient who aimed to continue living alone, was able to safely perform his goals using either a crutch or his self-propelled wheelchair. Shaun, who was to be discharged on bed rest for the majority of each day and whose only service was personal care, demonstrated his capacity to carry out ADLs.

Individualised carer education about patient assistance techniques was provided. Peter, the carer of Mary, was acquainted with his wife's supervision needs for all activities. He understood Mary's vulnerability when he was left alone with her in the ILU. For Fay, Sue's carer, education was focused on encouraging Sue to be more physically and mentally active.

The ILU trial helped Deborah, Leanne's carer, recognise her need for personal care assistance from a community service provider. Nursing staff showed Deborah how to assist Leanne with bed transfers at night. Janelle's husband Tim trialled initiatives such as a night alarm clock to manage Janelle's incontinence and learned to reheat meals in a microwave. Tim, who prior to the trial wanted no assistance at home, subsequently purchased a microwave and agreed to have a short-term package of community services.

Patricia, Henry's partner, stayed in the ILU with Henry and learned about Henry's changed eating requirements, reduced mobility and other aspects of his care. Henry had been very nervous about Patricia staying but found the time in the ILU with her helpful.

Discharge destination, mobility and support

Seventeen patients (72.3%) returned to their home. Three (13.6%) were temporarily discharged to a relative's home. One remained closer to the hospital for outpatient treatment, returning home once completed; another needed support while looking for accommodation closer to their relative; and the third was awaiting a vacancy in local transitional accommodation for patients with spinal cord injuries. One patient (4.5%) was discharged to a hospital closer to home to complete rehabilitation before returning home, and the other was discharged to a low-care residential aged care facility.

Figure 4.1 shows that 12 patients (54.5%) were discharged using a small frame to mobilise; five (22.7%) patients used a wheelchair (one was in self-propelled wheelchair pre-admission); three (13.4%) were using a walking stick and two patients (9.1%) were using crutches.

Family and community services at discharge

Upon discharge, all five carers in the study sample chose to continue caring for their relative, each of whom required more assistance than prior to admission. Two carers now had community assistance including personal care. Jane returned to her home because a relative chose to live with her.

Three patients (13.4%) aged over 65 were referred for a package of long-term assistance/care from community services. Three others (13.4%), aged over 70 years, were referred for a shorter term package of care which included rehabilitation to improve their mobility and home management with the aim of these patients not requiring long-term community assistance. One patient (4.5%) was referred for a six-week package of assistance. All packages of care included assistance with personal care, domestic chores (including shopping), and transport to health appointments.

Fifteen patients (68.2%) were transported home by a family member, with five patients (22.7%) having a discharge home visit with the occupational therapist to ensure equipment was set up properly at home. Two patients (9.1%) were transported home in a hire car or a taxi.

Thematic analysis: exploring the meaning

The following key issues emerged from a thematic analysis of ILU trial documentation. Each of these had implications for staff, patients and/or carers and the organisation.

Engagement and goal setting

A number of patients and carers did not share health staff concerns regarding their management at home despite the ILU trial rationale being discussed and consented to prior to commencement. These people had difficulty comprehending the trial's relevance. For example, both Gail and Gary ate the hospital meals during the trial rather than prepare their own meals. Ian and Gary who both had cognitive impairments were offended about having to demonstrate competency in the 'basic' ADL of meal preparation. They felt they were being treated like children. Ian and Jane anticipated their family or friends would be assisting them at home and did not see a need to perform some of the ADLs. Ian's friend, Monica, requested a reduction in ADL responsibility to align with the ADLs Ian performed pre-admission. Monica indicated an acceptance of Ian's pre-admission ADL function and declined an opportunity to improve his function.

However, with the exception of Jane, the other patients responded positively to reminders about the trial aims and to verbal prompts encouraging increased care and task responsibility. The ILU patients who seemed least able to accept a changed role were older and had experienced a bone fracture which had healed or was healing. They did not appear to view the injury as a significant event in their life and anticipated return home to life 'as normal' albeit now with a mobility aid.

For many of these patients a lack of familiarity with goal setting may have impacted on their ability to take ownership of their ADLs when initially relocated to the ILU (Barclay 2002). This resistance is something for staff to consider in relation to engagement, patient/carer education and preparation for the ILU experience. In this process particular attention is required for those patients with low MMSE scores.

In general, patients who actively engaged in the ILU trial were younger and had either permanent functional changes or complex injuries with an anticipated long recovery period following either a spinal cord injury or motor vehicle accident. These people recognised they would be discharged with significantly reduced function unlike other patients whose functional changes were less obvious to them but were of concern to health staff.

These findings appear to support the discharge planning statement: 'Older persons often underestimate how much assistance they will need (at least temporarily) after discharge from hospital. An older partner or carer may also underestimate how difficult it will be to provide care' (NSW Health 2007, p26). Miller et al. (2008) found that patients minimised the time it would take for them to recover and were unprepared for the degree of fatigue they experienced post-discharge.

ILU trials are an adjunct to staff provision of salient information to patients and carers about the realities of return home (Popejoy et al. 2009), by providing opportunity for patients and carers to experience an approximation of life at home, prior to discharge.

Our systematic, retrospective study also highlights a difference in understanding between some patients and healthcare teams as to the meaning and importance of promoting patient 'independence' (Barclay 2002, p7). Differences in emphasis could also reflect the impact of the institutional frame and the decision-making environment in which health staff conversations with patients and carers concerning ILU trials occur (Efraimsson et al. 2006; Moats 2006), an outcome of which can be disparity between staff, patient and carer expectations of each other. The patient's relinquishing of the sick role and the carer's regarding themselves as a partner in rehabilitation with the health team may be hard for some patients and carers to understand or accept in response to the expertise of the medical system.

'Home-like' environment

The relocation of patients from the more structured ward setting to the ILU, a room which provided support structures similar to those in the community and a physical environment enabling patients to behave 'as if they were home', appeared to facilitate, for some patients, recognition that an assessment of their ability to manage away from the hospital environment was taking place, resulting in greater engagement in the trial than if they had remained in their ward bed.

Some patients, however, rejected the analogy between the ILU environment and their own homes. One carer wanted to bring in kitchen appliances but was refused for occupational health and safety reasons. One patient became tired of waiting for a staff member to come on duty and prepared breakfast without initial supervision as originally agreed. Relatives of another patient complained that the furniture arrangement in the ILU made it harder for the patient to manage rather than helping them.

The continued provision of hospital meals to those with meal preparation tasks (in case the patient had become unwell and was unable to prepare a meal) proved to be confusing for several patients. These people chose to eat hospital meals rather than preparing their own. They went on to demonstrate meal preparation when reminded of this expected task.

Anxiety

Relocation to the ILU room proved to be an unsettling and anxiety-arousing experience for some older patients, even though the room was located in close vicinity to their prior hospital accommodation. One commented it was 'like going to prison'. Another described the experience as 'cruel, disgusting ... like being locked in a room with nothing in it.' Another patient indicated she felt lonely and requested relocation to a shared room on the ward at the completion of her trial.

Documentation

As is often the case, the conduct of this study based on available data revealed inadequate documentation of ILU admissions and processes.

In particular, routinely available data lacked specificity in relation to reasons for admission to the ILU, aims of the trial, trial commencement and completion dates, trial outcomes and impacts on discharge planning. Furthermore trial goals could have been more fully described and specified.

Early in the review period, an ILU schedule of proposed patient daily activities was developed for each patient. This has aided patients and staff to be clearer about daily routines. Currently it is difficult to determine from the documentation how often this schedule is referred to by staff and patients and whether this has made a difference to patient ownership of the activities of daily living (ADL) while in the ILU. The effective utilisation of this document offers an opportunity for further investigation.

Discussion

Clinical practice considerations

This CDM retrospective review demonstrates the value of time set aside for patients and carers to consider and discuss reasons for the recommended ILU trial. In particular, older patients who have difficulty appreciating the implications of their impairment may struggle with the trial's relevance. Patients and carers alike with impaired cognition also seem particularly vulnerable to distress or insult about requests to 'prove' their ability to master even the most basic tasks of living. Informed by the results of this study, a brochure explaining the ILU's purpose is being developed to assist with patient and carer understanding of the ILU resource in safe discharge planning.

Health staff, patients and carers each bring different world views, values, expectations, assumptions and understandings to conversations concerning care, assessment, treatment, goal setting and discharge planning (Wressle et al. 1999; McMurray et al. 2007). In the context of an ILU, staff may find it helpful to consider the values and objectives of the organisation, those of health staff, patients and carers, and the decision-making environment of the ward (Moats 2006). In particular, when patients and carers appear slow to accept an ILU trial recommendation, health staff should consider differences in understandings of concepts such as independence and patients as healthcare partners.

Education of patients, carers and new staff concerning goal setting in rehabilitation, and with particular regard to the ILU trials and ADL related goals, may improve understanding of goal setting in patient recovery (Wressle et al. 1999; Barclay 2002). It may also facilitate identification of goals that are meaningful to patients and their carers, thereby maintaining a client-centred approach (Wressle et al. 1999).

To date, patient feelings of anxiety and sense of isolation have been managed with a number of strategies including reminders of the trial reasons and agreed ADL tasks, reassurance, increased supervision and support in the first 24 hours. These strategies could be enhanced by early efforts at patient risk identification using anxiety-screening measures and counselling.

Obviously, staff rosters relevant to ILU patient tasks and goals are essential to successful ILU trials. This management and organisational issue may also contribute to the tensions between a 'hospital-like' and a 'home-like' environment and raises questions about the genuineness of viewing patients as partners in their treatment and recovery.

Clinical data mining: limitations and benefits

Clinical data mining is a 'practice-based, retrospective research strategy' (Epstein 2010, p71) which, while being labour intensive and time consuming, has enabled non-intrusive collection of available data concerning clinical practice and patient experience as reported by health staff. Emerging review insights relating to this sample of patient and carer ILU trial experiences now provides the rehabilitation team with significant data informing improvements to the ILU program. This includes communications, processes and documentation.

Although CDM has intrinsic methodological limitations, this study is limited by the small sample size. However, the team does consider the sample representative of the patient case mix admitted to the ward. It is also limited by the absence of some essential clinical data. Recent developments in information technology systems will enable further ILU review access to additional relevant data.

Other limitations of retrospective CDM of patient files have been outlined by Nilsson (2001). Of relevance to this sample is concern that the original documentation was conducted for clinical and not research purposes by many different staff over an extended (three-year) period; that is, the data can be questioned as to its reliability and consistency. Other events and issues in the patient admissions may not have been recorded, which, if recorded, may have informed the data analysis differently.

Nonetheless, this first ILU data-mining study has resulted in the construction of a new prospective dataset with the potential to enhance understanding of ILU rationales and processes and the development of a comprehensive patient profile of those who will benefit from a hospital-based ILU program. This makes possible future, prospective CDM studies with richer, more comprehensive and more reliable data.

Still, just the experience of meeting with ILU colleagues to talk about our practice has generated greater enthusiasm for the work we do. It has reinforced our belief in the uniqueness of each patient and patient system and the importance of being patient-centred in our approach.

Conclusions

The staff pre-review perception of an ILU as a beneficial resource assisting with successful and safe discharge planning for some patients is now considered accurate. The review indicated for the sample patients and carers an ILU trial assisted with discharge planning decision-making, in particular the type of support beneficial for both patients and carers. It also indicated that combination of age, cognition and injury type impact on patient responses and that assessment with regard to potential anxiety is essential to effective ILU processes. Despite these complexities the majority of patients and carers in this sample developed more confidence in their ability to manage on return home or requested additional support in order to successfully and safely return to community living.

Patient, carer and health staff understandings of concepts such as independence, agreement on how much the ILU represents being 'just like home', and patient and carer familiarity with goal setting should not be assumed but be part of the admission process and engagement with the ILU purpose. Recognising and addressing these differences in perception is core to effectively conducting health staff–patient–carer partnerships. Such partnerships will be further understood as data continues to be reviewed and accurate patient, carer and staff actions and responses are routinely recorded and considered by reflective health practitioners.

Acknowledgement is given to the members of the project team: C Bros (nursing unit manager), K Fischer (social worker), D Owen (social worker), A See (occupational therapist), J Swancott (social worker), A Thoroughgood (senior clinical dietitian), R Warner (occupational therapist).

References

Barclay L (2002). Exploring the factors that influence the goal setting process for occupational therapy intervention with an individual with spinal cord injury. *Australian Occupational Therapy Journal*, 49: 3–13.

Bauer M, Fitzgerald L, Haesler E & Manfrin M (2009). Hospital discharge planning for frail older people and their family: are we delivering best practice? A review of the evidence. *Journal of Clinical Nursing*, 18: 2539–46.

Becker MC, Abrams KS & Onder J (1974). Goal setting: a joint patient–staff method. *Archives of Physical Medicine and Rehabilitation*, 55: 87–89.

Black SJ, Brock KA, Kennedy G & Mackenzie M (2010). Is achievement of short-term goals a valid measure of patient progress in inpatient neurological rehabilitation? *Clinical Rehabilitation*, 24: 373–79.

Christianson CH (2005). Functional evaluation and management of self-care and other activities of daily living. In JA Delisa (Ed). *Physical medicine and rehabilitation: principles and practice* (pp975–1003). Philadelphia: Lippincott Williams and Wilkins.

Efraimsson E, Sandman PO, Hyden LC & Rasmussen BH (2006). How to get one's voice heard: the problems of a discharge planning conference. *Journal of Advanced Nursing*, 53(6): 646–55.

Epstein I (2010). *Clinical data-mining: integrating practice and research.* New York: Oxford University Press.

Gazewood JD (2009). Assessment of the older patient. In C Arenson, J Busby-Whitehead, K Brummel-Smith, JG O'Brien, MH Palmer & W Reichel (Eds). *Reichel's care of the elderly: clinical aspects of aging* (pp14–30). 6th edn. Cambridge: Cambridge University Press.

Glazier SR, Schuman J, Keltz E, Vally A & Galzier RH (2004). Taking the next steps in goal ascertainment: a prospective study of patient, team and family perspectives using a comprehensive standardised menu in a geriatric assessment and treatment unit. *Journal of the American Geriatrics Society,* 52: 284–89.

Haas JF (2005). Ethical issues in rehabilitation medicine. In JA Delisa (Ed). *Physical medicine and rehabilitation: principles and practice* (pp1085–97). Philadelphia: Lippincott Williams and Wilkins.

Hecker J (2002). Dementia and Alzheimer's disease. In RN Ratnaike (Ed). *Practical guide to geriatric medicine* (pp184–218). Sydney: The McGraw-Hill Companies.

Hutson C & Lichtiger E (2001). Mining clinical information in the utilisation of social services: practitioners inform themselves. *Social Work in Health Care,* 33(3): 153–61.

Manthorpe J (2009). Commentary on Bauer M, Fitzgerald L, Haesler E & Manfrin M (2009). Hospital discharge planning for frail older people and their family: are we delivering best practice? A review of the evidence. *Journal of Clinical Nursing,* 18: 2539–46, 18: 2676–77.

McMurray A, Johnson P, Wallis P, Patterson E & Griffiths S (2007). General surgical patients' perspectives of the adequacy and appropriateness of discharge planning to facilitate health decision-making at home. *Journal of Clinical Nursing,* 16: 1602–09.

Meier RH & Purtilo RB (1994). Ethical issues and the patient–provider relationship. *American Journal of Physical Medicine and Rehabilitation,* 73: 365–66.

Miller JM, Piacentine LB & Weiss M (2008). Coping difficulties after hospitalisation. *Clinical Nursing Research,* 17(4): 278–96.

Moats G (2006). Discharge decision-making with older people: the influence of the institutional environment. *Australian Occupational Therapy Journal*, 53: 107–16.

NSW Health (May 2007). Discharge planning: responsive standards. pp1–77.

Nilsson D (2001). Psycho-social problems faced by 'frequent flyers' in a pediatric diabetes unit. *Social Work in Health Care*, 33(3/4): 53–69.

Petersson P, Springett J & Blomqvist K (2009). Telling stories from everyday practice, an opportunity to see a bigger picture: a participatory action research project about developing discharge planning. *Health and Social Care in the Community*, 17(6): 548–56.

Popejoy LL, Moylan K & Galambos C (2009). A review of discharge planning research of older adults 1990–2008. *Western Journal of Nursing Research*, 31(7): 923–47.

Posenelli S, Joubert L, Power R, Vale S, Lewis A & Elliot R (2005). Managerial collaboration through allied health data-mining: the St Vincent's experience. *Journal of Social Work Research and Evaluation*, 6(2): 167–76.

Purtilo R & Meier RH (1993). Regulatory constraints and patient empowerment. *American Journal of Physical Medicine and Rehabilitation*, 72: 327–30.

Sivaraman Nair KP (2003). Life goals: the concept and its relevance to rehabilitation. *Clinical Rehabilitation*, 17: 192–202.

Wressle E, Oberg B & Henriksson C (1999). The rehabilitation process for the geriatric stroke patient: an exploratory study of goal setting and interventions. *Disability and Rehabilitation*, 21(2): 80–87.

Chapter 5

The hepatitis C treatment trifecta: alcohol, marijuana and mental illness

Gabrielle Murphy

Hepatitis C has the highest prevalence of all bloodborne viruses in Australia and is most often acquired by injecting drug use. Its treatment is lengthy, costly and psychologically demanding. This paper employs clinical data mining to examine the co-occurrence of three main risk factors – alcohol, marijuana and mental illness – in a hepatitis C pre-treatment population. Each of the three problems is known to complicate hepatitis C treatment compliance and success. The 'trifecta' combination of these factors together with socio-demographic risk factors creates contradictions and challenges for multidisciplinary treatment teams and highlights the vital importance of an individualised meaning-making approach in the pre-treatment and treatment phases.

Key words: drug and alcohol, viral hepatitis treatment, mental health issues, data mining

Understanding hepatitis C prevalence and treatment

The effective treatment of the hepatitis C virus (HCV) is a complex issue involving early detection, the identification and management of comorbidities, and the development of individualised treatment and supports. However, the issues of alcohol use and associated comorbidities of drug use and psychiatric illness complicate disease management, successful completion of treatment and the eradication of the virus (Loftis et al. 2006). Effective treatment of the combination of drug and alcohol abuse and associated mental health problems has been ironically dubbed the 'treatment trifecta' by some HCV clinicians.

HCV is a bloodborne virus which attacks the structure of the liver and leads to chronic liver disease in most cases, with an estimated 7% leading to cirrhosis if infected for more than 40 years. The symptoms of HCV are often mild and hard to differentiate from other general symptoms of ageing or poor lifestyle, yet it is the leading cause of liver transplantation in Australia (National Centre in HIV Epidemiology and Clinical Research 2010). The most frequently reported symptoms of HCV are fatigue, irritability, insomnia, nausea, muscle aches, headache, joint pain and abdominal discomfort (Hopwood 2003). HCV-related chronic liver disease, liver failure and liver transplant are extremely costly to the healthcare system, and as the population with HCV ages and disease severity worsens, the future medical needs of this population will increase.

Hepatitis C is the leading bloodborne virus affecting public health in Australia. In 2006, the estimated number of Australians living with hepatitis C was 284,000, an increase from the 2001 estimate of 210,000, which strongly suggests that the prevalence of HCV is increasing dramatically. In 2006, the Ministerial Advisory Committee on AIDS, Sexual Health and Hepatitis C estimated that at the present rate of 9700 new infections occurred annually and about 88% of new infections involved injecting drug users (IDU), (Ministerial Advisory Committee on AIDS, Sexual Health and Hepatitis C 2006). Despite these alarming statistics, recent studies indicate that HCV can be successfully eradicated in 50 to 80% of cases. However, the six or 12-month treatment regime presents a range of difficulties including the potential for physical, psychological and psychiatric complications (Paterson 2009).

HCV has six genotypes and more than 50 subtypes, which are often clustered in geographical regions around the world (Poynard 2002). In Australia, the majority of the genotypes are types 1–4 and each genotype has several subtypes (a, b and c). The most common types in Australia are 1 (55%) and 3 (35%) (Ministerial Advisory Committee on AIDS, Sexual Health and Hepatitis C 2006). While the various types and subtypes do not actually affect the rate of disease progression, they do alter treatment success rates and therefore affect long-term health implications (Poynard 2002). This may be due to subtle differences in the virus as it has mutated, making some genotypes more susceptible to eradication with the current treatment regime.

The current standard therapy involves the self-injected sub-cutaneous use of pegylated (long-acting) Interferon once per week, and twice-daily Ribavirin in tablet form (Peg-IFN and RBV) and is often referred to as combination therapy. This regime continues for 24 or 48 weeks, depending on various biological and disease factors. Success rates are variable – up to 80% success for types 2 and 3 with 24 weeks of treatment, but as little as 50% success for types 1 and 4 and those with cirrhosis with 48-week treatment.

In addition to varied success rates, the treatment side-effect profile is formidable. Thus, Loftis et al. comment: 'It is well accepted that IFN (Interferon) can cause significant neuropsychiatric adverse effects, including symptoms of depression, fatigue, anxiety, irritability, sexual dysfunction, anorexia, hypersomnia, anhedonia, psychomotor retardation, impaired concentration, apathy and confusion' (Loftis et al. 2006, p159). In addition, discontinued or unsuccessful therapy has been shown to reduce the efficacy of second or subsequent treatment attempts.

Under the Australian Government's Pharmeceutical Benefits Scheme – Specialised Drugs Scheme (PBS – S100), the cost of the drugs used in the first attempt are essentially free. Access to a second course of treatment is also covered under the PBS, but is bound by stricter management protocols, reflecting the reality that a second course of treatment is much less likely to be successful if the first attempt failed. Recent reports indicate that as few as 2% of HCV-positive patients receive treatment each year, but recommend at least a tripling of the numbers of people accessing combination therapy in order to minimise the social and medical impact of this disease in the future (Ministerial Advisory Committee on AIDS, Sexual Health and Hepatitis C 2006).

The most commonly cited reason for the discontinuation of hepatitis C treatment is intolerance of the psychiatric side effects, such as depression, in up to 30% of treatment populations (Hopwood et al.

2006). At an estimated cost to the PBS of $10,000 per six-month course for the medication alone, with additional cost for the clinician time and pathology tests borne by Medicare, the successful completion of therapy at first attempt is a highly prized goal for doctors, patients and funding bodies alike. Anything that helps promote and predict positive treatment outcomes is highly valued. Likewise, identifying those most at risk of treatment failure or premature discontinuation are of great interest to hepatitis treatment teams, program administrators and policymakers alike.

In Australia as in most Western industrialised countries, large proportions of the general population are exposed to recreational marijuana, and the public view it as a 'soft' or 'natural' drug, with some medicinal benefits. Hence, in the screening phase leading up to treatment, HCV-positive patients are more likely to admit marijuana use, but less likely to admit injecting drug use due to its socially unacceptable associations with criminality. However, the majority of new and existing cases of HCV involve injecting drug use (IDU) and in this population, not surprisingly, the prevalence of psychiatric co-morbidity is high (Loftis et al. 2006). Marijuana has also been strongly associated with psychiatric illness and its use in Australia is often linked with other illicit drug use in the 'at risk' population for HCV infection. Thus, there are also strong associations between psychiatric illness, substance use disorder and HCV. In the HCV-positive population, continued alcohol intake is an added complication as it progresses liver disease and also decreases the response to combination therapy (Loftis et al. 2006).

This study 'mines' available data concerning HCV-positive patients who presented to the Liver Treatment Clinic of John Hunter Hospital (JHH), a large tertiary referral hospital in Newcastle, NSW, Australia. This study focuses on the use of marijuana instead of injecting drug use due to the number of patients who disclosed marijuana use in the screening phase, but who denied injecting drug use. The study aims to identify those patients with high alcohol, marijuana, mental illness and other demographic factors which may put them at risk of treatment failure or discontinuation.

Literature review

Australian drug and alcohol usage data suggest that 35% of Australians drink alcohol at levels considered risky for short-term harm (binge drinking) and 10% at levels of high risk for long-term harm. Marijuana is the most common illicit drug used in Australia, with 34% of the population having used it in their lifetime. Alcohol is the most common principal drug of concern in those seeking treatment for addiction (37%) followed by marijuana (23%) and heroin (17%). Depression (68%) and anxiety (38%) were the most common mental health problems for which injecting drug users (IDU) sought assistance (Australian Institute of Health and Welfare 2006).

In the field of mental health and psychiatry, marijuana has been associated with higher rates of psychotic illness, particularly schizophrenia. Research on marijuana consumption has also identified some positive uses – for example, as an alternative to medication to reduce nausea, improve appetite, reduce aches and pains and improve sleep, and ironically to improve adherence to HCV treatment. However, marijuana use has also been strongly linked to liver fibrosis (a breakdown of healthy tissue and replacement by less functional fibrous tissue) and steatosis (fatty build-up around liver) both of which are associated with a decrease in success rates of HCV treatment (Fisher et al. 2006).

In several studies cited by Verdoux, marijuana use was strongly associated with both passive symptoms of psychosis (perceptual anomalies and magical/paranoid ideation) and negative symptoms (physical and social anhedonia or depressed mood). These studies suggest that marijuana use is an independent risk factor for the onset of psychosis, most marked in people with an established vulnerability for psychosis based on genetic and familial factors (Verdoux 2004).

The link between marijuana use and depression is still not firmly established. In a review of literature, Degenhardt et al. reported that an Australian study found those who use cannabis most heavily were also more likely to meet the *Diagnostic and statistical manual of mental disorders: 4th edition (DSM-IV)* mood disorder criteria by a rate of two to three times. However, this association is still unclear, as other studies with differing methodology have not found this link as clearly (Degenhardt et al. 2004).

In a prospective study of 293 veterans in a HCV treatment centre in Oregon, US, Fireman et al. found that 93% reported current or past history of at least one psychiatric or substance use disorder and 73% reported two or more disorders. Depression was found in 81% of this population and alcohol or other substance use disorder in 58% (Fireman et al. 2005).

Loftis et al. (2006) discussed trimorbidity and reported that 'the majority of new and existing cases of HCV are related to injecting drug use and, in this population, the prevalence of psychiatric comorbidity is high' (Loftis et al. 2006, p156). They go on to report that the relationship between alcohol use and HCV-related progression of liver disease is synergistic, with those with heavier alcohol consumption (i.e. >30 g/day) at higher risk of developing cirrhosis and fibrosis and a lower survival rate compared to patients who drink <30 g/day, where one standard drink contains 10 g alcohol. These HCV researchers also conclude that alcohol users (within the last 12 months) have a higher rate of HCV treatment discontinuation compared with non-users.

Further to this, Fisher et al. report that studies found that HCV treatment patients have significantly lower quality of life scores than general populations (Fischer et al. 2006). In a large review of veterans in a US-wide survey, Lim et al. found that health-related quality of life was significantly reduced in HCV-positive veterans not seeking treatment. Furthermore they were also much more likely to have alcohol dependence and depression. These studies suggest that the quality of life of those living with HCV is compromised and the combination treatment further reduces quality of life for the treatment period (Lim et al. 2006).

These treatment problems are not unique to Australia. In a study of young IDUs in the US, Costenbader et al. (2007) reported that 25% of heroin users entering drug and alcohol treatment in 2002 reported use of alcohol as a secondary substance, indicating that significant numbers of people at high risk of acquiring HCV are also at risk of alcohol misuse. Costenbader also points out that while alcohol has been consistently linked to depression in the literature, it has not been established whether those who are depressed use alcohol to self-medicate or whether use of alcohol leads to depression (Costenbader et al. 2007). This question suggests that much is still to be learned about the relationships between alcohol and depression. Of course, similar questions can be raised about marijuana use and its link to depression and other psychiatric illness.

A cross-sectional study of 65 patients on IFN treatment in a hepatology clinic in the mid-western US, conducted by Zickmund and colleagues, combined semi-structured interviews and the self-administered Hospital Anxiety and Depression Scale (HADS) tool to help establish current anxiety and depressive symptoms. This study showed that higher anxiety and depression subscales on the HADS were associated with greater reported difficulties with treatment. In fact, highly anxious and depressed patients reported that treatment side effects were more troubling than the symptoms of the underlying disease itself. Patients in general reported that the principle of complete abstinence from alcohol advised by most treatment centres caused social isolation. Zickmund and colleagues comment:

> They struggled with a desire for a social drink and lamented the loss of social contact that abstinence had brought. In addition, a break from these habits often also meant a break from family and friends, further reducing the ability to cope with treatment (Zickmund et al. 2006, p385).

This study highlights the importance of even minimal alcohol use in maintaining social contact for some people, the loss of which could be keenly felt at a time when social support is essential to treatment completion and success.

Psychiatric illness in HCV treatment populations is an area of study dominated by investigations into depression with little research into anxiety. In a study of 90 patients in a tertiary treatment centre in Dublin, Golden and colleagues reported that 24% of participants had an anxiety disorder, when interviewed by a psychiatrist using DSM-IV criteria. A further 8% qualified for an anxiety and depression disorder. In addition, 86% of those with anxiety had the disorder diagnosed for the first time in the Dublin study, suggesting anxiety is largely under-identified in the HCV population (Golden et al. 2005).

In combination, the foregoing studies highlight the complexity of the link between alcohol use, marijuana, mental illness and HCV. The effective treatment of HCV relies heavily on the timely identification of mental health problems, alcohol use and drug use, particularly marijuana due to its link to psychosis and possible depression. When working with HCV, the patient group is often vulnerable to substance use disorders and psychiatric illness, making it essential for all team members to work in an inclusive, supportive and educative way to maximise the patients' chances of gaining access to and completing treatment. The presence of a 'trifecta' of alcohol, marijuana and mental illness is likely to appear in a significant proportion of a treatment population. This requires service providers to understand this complex combination of factors in local populations and to develop clear guidelines and protocols in order to maximise effective assessment and treatment.

Aims of the study

The study aimed in the first instance to examine relationships between anxiety and depression, marijuana and alcohol use in the context of preparation for hepatitis C treatment at the JHH clinic. These findings were then used to improve the quality of pre-treatment assessment and on-treatment care, so that those who undertake treatment have the greatest chance of completing treatment and re-starting life free of HCV.

Informing these aims were participating clinicians' wish to know more about the often silent factors working for and against the treatment success, mainly current alcohol intake, marijuana and their links to anxiety and depression. Such knowledge would better inform clinicians working in these settings to develop individualised treatment programs, using combinations of medications such as anti-depressants, individual support through counselling and referral to drug and alcohol services or group programs such as Alcoholics Anonymous. To make maximum use of both costly and arduous treatment protocols, it is essential to target those patients at higher risk of treatment-related psychiatric complications before they become significantly symptomatic and put treatment continuation at risk. An Ethics Waiver was obtained from the Hunter Research Ethics Committee for the completion of the project as a 'clinical data-mining' (CDM) project (Epstein 2010).

Organisational context

John Hunter Hospital is a 600-bed tertiary referral hospital located in Newcastle 200 kilometres north of Sydney, NSW, Australia. The Outpatient Viral Hepatitis Service is a multidisciplinary team of doctors, nurse practitioner, clinical nurse specialist, clinical trials coordinator and social worker. The team assesses approximately 275 patients annually and has treated an average of 90 with combination Interferon/Ribavirin medication each year over the last six years. The referral pathway for accessing treatment includes a mandatory assessment by nurse practitioner, medical specialist and social worker prior to establishing patients' suitability for the treatment. The multidisciplinary team take this assessment phase seriously due to the long commitment demanded on each patient and the potential for serious psychiatric and physical side effects.

Methodology

This study is a retrospective CDM study, using data routinely gathered from patients during semi-structured social work interviews. All social work assessments conducted since 2001 have used a standard assessment form to gather pertinent psychosocial details on past alcohol, current alcohol and current marijuana use. This assessment included completion of the Hospital Anxiety and Depression Scale (HADS). The data collected in the assessment was then transferred on to a Microsoft Access database. Several steps toward de-identification of data were undertaken such as the removal of names, addresses and the conversion of date of birth into an age and incomplete records removed.

During the interviews, the patient was asked all alcohol-related questions in terms of number and types of drinks they had per week. Answers to these questions were entered into a table on the assessment form which converted drink types and amounts into a 'grams of alcohol per week' format, where one standard drink equated to 10 g of alcohol. In this manner, 'six schooners of beer' was calculated as six times 16 g of alcohol or 96 g. The National Health and Medical Research Council (NHMRC) states that one standard drink (10 g of alcohol) is equivalent to one middy of full strength beer (285 ml), a small glass of wine (100 ml) or one nip of spirits(30 ml) (Australian Guidelines to Reduce Health Risks from Drinking Alcohol 2009).

It is important to acknowledge the likelihood of underestimation of alcohol and drug use in self-report scales as used in this study. True consumption figures might be significantly higher than what is reported here. This problem is not unique, however, to CDM studies.

When interpreting tables for 'risk', it is important to consider that 'risky' drinking (as outlined by the NHMRC) refers to healthy people. Anyone with HCV or other chronic liver disease is at much higher risk than a healthy person of developing medical complications from even moderate alcohol consumption. Therefore 'risk' in healthy populations does not directly correspond with 'risk' in liver-compromised patients. With this in mind, the social worker and JHH drug and alcohol service developed an empirically based classification system using patient-reported grams of alcohol consumed per week (Table 5.1) which was used in the social work assessment to categorise relative risk.

Table 5.1: Alcohol intake classification system

Rating	Description
0	No alcohol at all, a 'non-drinker'
1	Low risk alcohol use, social drinker, 0–50 g alcohol per week (or up to 5 standard drinks)
2	Moderate alcohol risk, regular drinker 51–100 g alcohol per week (6 to 10 standard drinks)
3	High risk alcohol use, heavy drinker more than 100 g/week (more than 10 standard drinks per week)

Sample

The sample studied in this report were patients who attended a one-hour, in-depth psychosocial assessment with the viral hepatitis social worker. The data originated between 2002 and 2008. In this period a total of 512 patients were assessed and psychosocial data were entered onto a computerised database. Because the HADS instrument was introduced as a screening tool in mid-2003, for the purposes of this CDM study, cases with complete HADS scores and full drug and alcohol histories reduced the number that could be systematically examined to 289.

Data sources and collection process

The data examined here was gathered at a routine and compulsory psychosocial assessment at the Liver Clinic to establish the patient's stability and ultimate suitability for entry onto the combination therapy program. The data includes basic demographic data such as age, gender, marital status as well as employment, income source and type of housing. Specific data related to hepatitis C was gathered, namely the main risk factors for HCV, length of time since diagnosis, method of diagnosis and patterns of disclosure of HCV status. General health data which has particular relevance to HCV treatment was also included, namely drug and alcohol history and current intake, mental health history and the patient's scores on the Hospital Anxiety and Depression Scale (HADS).

The HADS is a brief, easily administered, 14-point scale assessing anxiety and depression with no questions about the physical manifestations of any medical conditions and is structured around seven anxiety- and seven depression-related questions. It is used widely internationally and has been extensively tested for validity and reliability (Bjelland et al. 2002). It is easy to administer for low literacy, easy to score and well received by clients and workers alike. The HADS is recommended for use in clinical settings when screening for depression and anxiety and their severity. It effectively demonstrates change over time and can be used in conjunction with other tools. It was designed for each subscale to be scored and interpreted separately, not interpreted as a total score. For use in this setting, the HCV team in conjunction with the JHH Psychiatry Liaison Service (PLS) created a guideline for 'recommended action' based on the patient's scores on the HADS as outlined in Table 5.2.

Table 5.2: Reference range for interpretation of the HADS

Score range	Likely interpretation	Recommended action
0–7 on either scale	No current anxiety or depression symptoms	No action
8–11 on either scale	Possible anxiety or depression symptoms	Monitor symptoms, provide support, discuss management strategies
12 or above on either scale	Probable anxiety or depression symptoms	Discuss symptoms, refer to general practitioner or Psychiatry Liaison Service for more thorough assessment

Results

A total of 289 patients with full demographic, alcohol and HADS score were identified from a total pool of 512 patients assessed by the social worker between 2003 and 2008. The past and current rates of alcohol use represented in Figure 5.1 show that a vast majority of patients do make significant changes to their alcohol intake levels in the weeks or months leading up to treatment. This is suggested by the fact that 69 (23%) of patients reported past abstinence but a further 132 (46%) reported current abstinence. This result is reinforced by the number of people who report *past* heavy alcohol use is 100 (34%) but this drops to 34 (12%) for *current* heavy alcohol use. This data suggests that many heavy drinkers are able to report a successful shift from heavy use to abstinence leading up to treatment, while other heavy drinkers shift towards moderate intake or social intake rather than complete abstinence. However, when treatment teams are advocating complete abstinence leading up to and while on treatment, this data suggests that more than half of the patients are still drinking some alcohol, with 23% still drinking more than 50 g/week. The data also indicate that past low or social alcohol use (27%) and moderate use (14%) remain relatively unchanged leading up to HCV treatment (31% and 11% respectively).

Figure 5.1: Self-reported previous and current alcohol use in patients seeking HCV treatment.

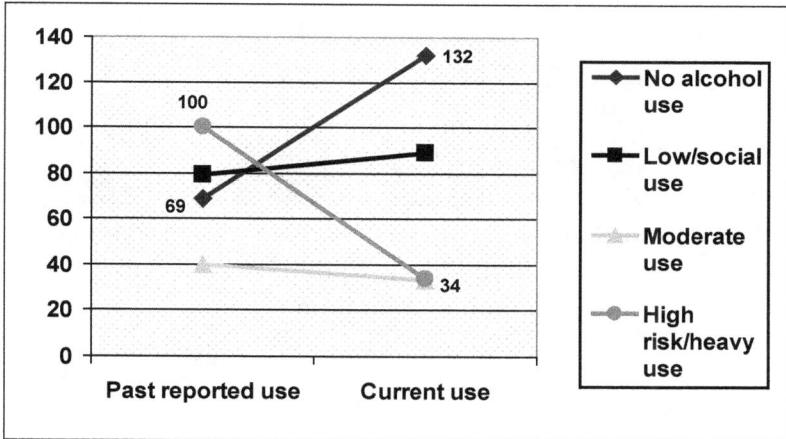

When investigating links between alcohol and psychiatric illness, this study showed that anxiety is a much more common problem than depression in the JHH population. As demonstrated in Figure 5.2 high levels of anxiety (HADS scores of 12 or more on anxiety subscale) are similar through the three lower levels of risk (15%, 15%, 12%) but then peak at the 'high alcohol' risk level at 23%. In contrast, high levels of depression (HADS score of 12 or more on the depression subscale) are similar across the 'none', 'low' and 'moderate' alcohol risk categories (4%, 5%, 6%).

These data indicate that there is a trend between heavy alcohol use and increasing risk for anxiety and depression at almost double the rate of the moderate alcohol users. The cumulative effect of high alcohol use indicates that 32% of heavy alcohol users have high risks for anxiety or depression symptoms leading up to treatment.

Figure 5.2: Alcohol 'risk' levels and high scores on the HADS subscales for anxiety and depression.

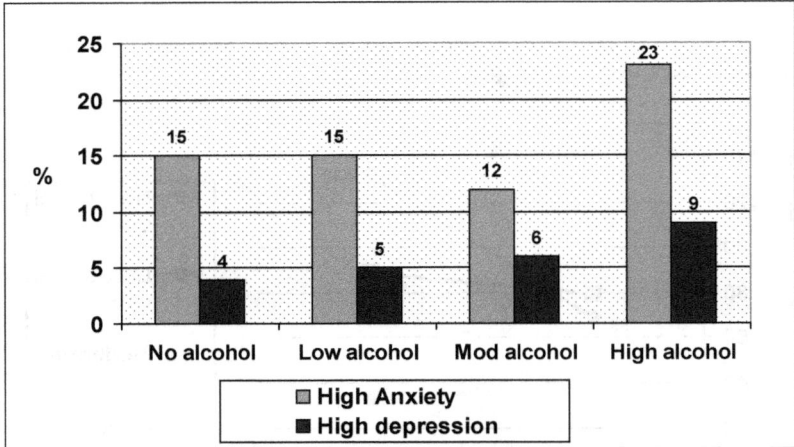

Table 5.3: Marijuana use by alcohol risk factor (%).

	No alcohol%	Low-risk alcohol% (0–50 g/ week)	Moderate risk alcohol% (51–100 g/ week)	High-risk alcohol% (100 g+/ week)
No marijuana	70	62	54	55
Social/ occasional marijuana	11	20	12	8
Regular marijuana	9	5	9	24
Heavy/daily marijuana	10	12	24	11

The high anxiety levels among this population (average of 15% in this population) are higher than the estimated 10% of Australian people who experience some type of anxiety disorder in any one year (Beyond Blue n.d.).

As marijuana use is strongly associated with psychiatric illness, especially psychosis and growing evidence for depression, the recent use of this drug was analysed according to the current reported levels of alcohol use.

Table 5.3 shows that while the bulk of patients fit into the 'none' or 'low' categories for both alcohol and marijuana (81% and 82% combined), more than a third of patients who smoked marijuana regularly or heavily also consumed alcohol at moderate or high-risk levels. This suggests that the combination of heavy alcohol use, which affects treatment success rates, and regular or heavy marijuana use, which is linked to mental illness and can result in early treatment cessation, occurs at dangerous levels in 23% of this group.

Overall, this data indicates that significant anxiety and depression symptoms occur in much of the treatment population and that risky alcohol use and regular or heavy marijuana use is also found in significant numbers of this pre-treatment population.

To provide a greater depth of understanding of the life-risk factors associated with the 'treatment trifecta', a smaller subset of the data was examined, looking at the socio-demographic factors or characteristics of those patients who were reporting high alcohol use at initial social work assessment. This group initially numbered more than 30, but missing data resulted in a group of 23 patients. When examined, a series of 12 possible demographic or life-risk factors became evident. These are reported in Table 5.4.

When looking at these socio-demographics as possible risk factors that may further stress or complicate the lives of people already at high risk of not completing the treatment program, 60% of these 23 people had five or more factors, with three individuals registering eight factors.

Age and gender also played an important role in this group, with the average age being 42 years (range 26–58 years). When gender was considered, the men tended to be older (average 43 years, range

26–58) while women were younger (average 40 years, range 30–44). Interestingly, income source was not as clear a risk factor as anticipated, with as many high alcohol drinkers on the Disability Support Pension (DSP) as had salary or wages as their main income source.

Table 5.4: Demographic and life-risk factors in the high alcohol subset.

Life-Risk Factor	% of clients in high alcohol use subset
Male gender	69
Private rental accommodation	56
Unemployed	52
Injecting drug use as primary risk factor for HCV	52
Married or defacto relationship	43
Heavy or regular marijuana use	39
Living with family	39
Diagnosed for between 1 and 5 years	39
History of depression	39
Income source of Government Disability Support Pension	30
High anxiety (current)	26
High depression (current)	13

Discussion

HCV, alcohol and treatment efficacy

Patients receiving a HCV diagnosis are generally counselled by their physicians to abstain from drinking alcohol in order that they avert further liver damage. Some patients were in the unfortunate position of receiving their HCV diagnosis many years after they acquired the disease, and were unaware of the damage their alcohol use was having on their liver. Despite significant education about existing liver damage and detrimental effects on treatment outcome, a significant number of people are unable or unwilling to alter their alcohol use.

The population in this study usually had a minimum of four contacts with a healthcare worker or professional prior to assessment from the social worker. These professionals typically include a general practitioner for diagnosis and referral, nurse practitioner for first-line clinical triage and hepatologist/immunology and infectious disease specialist for medical review. In many cases, the contacts with healthcare workers could number over 10, due to the length of time since diagnosis and time spent in a specialist's care prior to referral to treatment services. Referral to treatment is at the specialist's discretion, and usually determined by factors such as blood markers, severity of symptoms and the patient's willingness to undertake treatment. Despite these contacts, many patients report little understanding of the reasons why alcohol abstinence is advised, in terms of the basic mechanisms of liver injury with hepatitis C and alcohol together. Whether this is due to the patient not being told, or being told in terms that they cannot understand, is not known. However, it is of great concern that many patients do not seem to be fully aware of the synergistic relationship between alcohol and worsening liver disease and therefore choices about alcohol intake are not based on being fully cognisant of the dangers. Many patients report an understanding that alcohol use must end when treatment begins, but not why it must end nor strategies for how this might be managed. This poor understanding leads to questions about the efficacy of current education regarding alcohol use with HCV, and suggests that further investigation needs to be completed to develop more effective education and intervention strategies for the high-risk alcohol users. These strategies may include further research to understand the meaning of the disease, the process of education messages delivery and the understanding of the treatment response.

Depression

The literature indicates alcohol has been linked to depression although it has not been established whether those who are depressed use alcohol to self-medicate or whether use of alcohol leads to depression (Costenbader et al. 2007). In this study, a link between depression and alcohol is evident, although the degree to which it is linked is still tenuous. The most pressing issue for pre-existing depression is the likelihood of treatment-induced depression occurring during combination therapy (Paterson 2009). While combination therapy-induced depression can occur in people with no history of depression, the treatment is also likely to cause an exacerbation of mild or moderate depression, requiring a pharmacotherapy intervention such as an antidepressant, or in severe cases, a cessation of treatment. In this study, the frequency of depression in the pre-treatment population is not overtly worrisome, but the risk of depression occurring in previously well patients, or a worsening of even mild depression, suggests that very close assessment prior to and throughout treatment should be a priority.

Anxiety

Interferon (IFN) therapy is well documented to be a cause of anxiety symptoms and has been noted to be one reason for the premature discontinuation of treatment. In this study the very strong association between anxiety and moderate and high alcohol use is of great concern, because of the risk of alcohol being used as a self-medication, causing ongoing liver damage, or for the worsening of anxiety symptoms if alcohol use is stopped while on treatment. All these scenarios are of concern – more severe liver disease, more severe anxiety, early treatment discontinuation or treatment failure. This outcome is a very significant issue for patients and workers alike. Early identification and management of symptoms such as anxiety are essential to increase the completion rates of treatment and ultimately improve the rates of viral clearance and quality of life of the patient group.

Marijuana

Statistics on drug use in Australia (Australian Institute of Health and Welfare 2006) indicate that marijuana is the most common illicit drug used in Australia with 11% of the population having used it in the last 12 months. The data in the current study found that almost 34% of the pre-treatment population used marijuana more than 'occasionally', with 13% using marijuana in a heavy manner (i.e. at least once daily). This, in conjunction with an expected level of under-reporting, suggests that marijuana use in the HCV-positive population is a much larger issue than in the general population. When marijuana use is combined with risks for steatosis (fatty build up around liver), psychosis, depression and other mental health issues, the heavy marijuana smoking group, although a small number within the HCV population, is a group very vulnerable to psychiatric complications in their lifetime, and while on treatment have reduced chances of viral clearance.

Life-risk factors

The identification of a series of life-risk factors linked with high alcohol use in this population provides some direction for clinicians when preparing patients for treatment. While some of the life-risk factors identified, such as low income, unemployment, inadequate housing and lack of social support, are all intricately linked to poorer health status and increased likelihood of mental illness (Australian Institute of Health and Welfare 2010, p80), other factors are surprising. For example, 43% of patients drinking heavily were in a married or defacto relationship, indicating the existence of some form of social connection and intimate support and 30% had salary or wages as main income source, indicating an ability to maintain employment. These findings challenge the picture many clinicians have of an unemployed, financially limited, socially isolated single man as a candidate for treatment complications. The 'treatment trifecta' presents a genuine set of risk factors for clinicians; however, the person experiencing the 'trifecta' is just as likely to experience one or a series of positive factors, such as marriage or employment, requiring the clinician to be considering both 'risk' and resilience factors in the pre-treatment and treatment setting.

This study indicates the prevalence of a treatment trifecta in the HCV population. However, it also indicates that this comorbid population is not confined to the type of financially limited, socially isolated, vulnerable single man. Those at risk of a treatment trifecta could be male or female, be in a stable relationship, have stable accommodation and work for a living. This surprise finding indicates the need for the HCV treatment team to be alert for the trifecta across the entire clinic population and to be ready to work on an uniquely individualised and detailed holistic support process that engages each person's risk factors and strengths, the meaning they make of the diagnosis and treatment, and support planning to enable them to remain on treatment during their first attempt.

Limitations

This study is limited by the risk that the role of the social worker is seen as a 'gatekeeper', controlling access to a much-desired treatment, which may discourage full and uninhibited disclosure about some aspects of a patient's medical, social or psychiatric past. The patient may fear that truthful answers to questions about drugs, alcohol or mental health issues may put them in 'unfavourable' light with the treatment team or make them ineligible. A further limitation is the reliability of self-reported drug and alcohol measures, particularly in the context of answers being linked to the patients' eligibility for treatment. Likewise, validity studies using the HADS in the HCV population have not been widely examined; however, it is designed and widely validated for use in outpatient populations, as in this study.

The social worker endeavoured to work in a collaborative way with the client and encourage the transfer of accurate information to assist all healthcare staff to provide the best and custom-made care, specific to the needs of the individual. However, the accuracy of any information provided by individuals in this study will vary according to issues such as fear of stigma, memory, sense of wellbeing and a patient's level of understanding.

A specific limitation is present with the data collection method in the semi-structured interviews. When interviewing patients about their drug and alcohol use, information was sought about 'past alcohol use' and 'current alcohol/marijuana use' with no specific formula for specifying what 'past' or 'current' meant. However, in the context of a treatment interview, the social worker has assumed that 'past' meant the time between 'receiving HCV diagnosis' and 'seeking treatment for HCV'. For many patients, this timeframe is quite quick (six months between initial diagnosis and treatment interview) while for others this may be many years.

For the purposes of the database, no data was gathered as to specific cultural issues such as Aboriginal or Torres Strait Islander background, sexual orientation or English as a second language issues. This data is available to the workers in the health system through the health computer infrastructure, but was not specifically sought at social work interview. Access to this type of information may assist in the future identification of more vulnerable groups in society and their needs.

Conclusions

This CDM study provides data-driven insight into the patterns of alcohol and marijuana use in the pre-treatment population, and their links to anxiety and depression. It demonstrates that while most patients do make changes to alcohol consumption prior to starting treatment, a significant proportion of people still drink alcohol at high-risk levels despite education and support, putting their treatment success at risk. While depression continues to be one of the most troubling issues for early treatment cessation, the issues of high anxiety are a much more significant factor in the pre-treatment population. Likewise, while heavy marijuana use is an issue for only a small group of people in this study, the risk factors linked to its use, both psychiatrically and regarding treatment efficacy, mean marijuana use is of great concern for the treating teams.

The need for good client–clinician relationships resulting in frank and honest discussions of drug and alcohol and mental health backgrounds, as well as transparent assessment pathways, are essential for the successful engagement and treatment of this vulnerable group. An individualised assessment and management approach for patients preparing for treatment should be a 'best practice' target. Although somewhat time-intensive, the use of a variety of clinicians, tools and intervention modalities is likely to assist in the early identification of mental health and drug and alcohol issues, and appropriate management approaches on an individualised basis. This strategy may lead to better adherence to treatment, better rates of completion and ultimately better clearance rates of the virus, leading to higher quality of life in people who underwent the treatment.

Unfortunately, in the HCV 'treatment trifecta', relatively few patients win the race. This combination increases the risk of psychological symptoms during treatment, worsens overall liver health, reduces treatment success rates and leads to higher risks for liver complications such as cirrhosis and liver failure. However, an inclusive, supportive and educative approach to the needs of this vulnerable group may ameliorate the trifecta's risk factors and make a substantial difference in this group's longevity and quality of life.

Acknowledgements:

The author would like to thank the Consortium for Social and Policy Research at the National Centre in HIV Social Research for support of a research capacity building internship. She also thanks the team at the JHH Liver Treatment Clinic for their support over the last nine years, particularly Tracey Jones, Liz Ianna, Nadine Leembruggen, Carla Silva and Dr Brian Hughes, as well as Fran Hodgson and the JHH Social Work Department. The support of Ros Giles and Anne Vertigan is also highly valued and immensely appreciated.

References

Australian Institute of Health and Welfare (2010). *Australia's Health 2010*. Australia's Health series no. 12. cat. no. AUS 122. Canberra: Australian Institute of Health and Welfare.

Australian Institute of Health and Welfare (2006). *Statistics on drug use in Australia 2006*. Canberra: Australian Government Department of Health and Ageing.

Beyond Blue (n.d.). Anxiety disorders factsheet. Beyond Blue: The National Depression Initiative. [Online]. Available: www.beyondblue.org.au/index. aspx?link_id=90 [Accessed 10 August 2010].

Bjelland I, Dahl A, Haug T & Neckelmann D (2002). The validity of the Hospital Anxiety and Depression Scale: an updated literature review. *Journal of Psychosomatic Research*, 52(2): 69–77.

Costenbader E, Zule W & Coomes C (2007). The impact of illicit drug use and harmful drinking in quality of life among injection drug users at high risk for hepatitis C infection. *Drug and Alcohol Dependence*, 89(2–3): 251–58.

Degenhardt L, Hall W, Lynskey M, Coffey C & Patton G (2004). The association between cannabis use and depression: a review of the evidence. In D Castle & R Murray (Eds). *Marijuana and madness: psychiatry and neurobiology* (pp54–74). New York: Cambridge University Press.

Epstein I (2010). *Clinical data-mining: integrating practice and research*. New York: Oxford University Press.

Fireman M, Indest D, Blackwell A, Whitehead A & Hauser P (2005). Addressing trimorbidity (hepatitis C, psychiatric disorders and substance use): the importance of routine mental health screening as a component of a comanagement model of care. *Clinical Infectious Diseases,* 40: S286–91.

Fisher B, Reimer J, Firestone M, Kalousek K, Rehm J & Heathcate J (2006). Treatment for hepatitis C virus and cannabis use in illicit drug user patients: implications and questions. *European Journal of Gastroenterology and Hepatology*, 18: 1039–42.

Golden J, O'Dwyer A & Conroy R (2005). Depression and anxiety in patients with hepatitis C: prevalence, detection rates and risk factors. *General Hospital Psychiatry*, 27: 431–38.

Hopwood M (2003). New treatment for hepatitis C infection. *Social research briefs* 3. [Online]. Available: nchsr.arts.unsw.edu.au/media/File/SRB03.pdf [Accessed 25 March 2011].

Hopwood M, Treloar C & Redsull L (2006). *Experiences of hepatitis C treatment and its management: what some patients and health professionals say* (Monograph 4/2006). Sydney: National Centre in HIV Social Research, University of New South Wales.

Lim J, Cronkite R, Goldstein M & Cheung R (2006). The impact of chronic hepatitis C and comorbid psychiatric illness on health-related quality of life. *Journal of Clinical Gastroenterology*, 40(6): 528–34.

Loftis J, Matthews A & Hauser P (2006). Psychiatric and substance use disorders in individuals with hepatitis C: epidemiology and management. *Drugs*, 66 (2): 155–74.

Ministerial Advisory Committee on AIDS, Sexual Health and Hepatitis C Sub-committee (2006). Hepatitis C virus projections working group: estimates and projections of the hepatitis C virus epidemic in Australia 2006. Department of Health and Ageing. [Online]. Available: www.health.gov.au/internet/publications/publishing.nsf/Content/phd-hepc-estimates-project-06-l [Accessed 25 March 2011].

National Centre in HIV Epidemiology and Clinical Research (2010). *Epidemiological and economic impact of potential increased hepatitis C treatment uptake in Australia.* Sydney: NCHECR, University of New South Wales.

National Health and Medical Research Council (2009). *Australian guidelines to reduce health risks from drinking alcohol.* Canberra: National Centre in HIV Social Research National Health and Medical Research Council.

Paterson BL (2009). Barriers to starting and completing hepatitis C treatment. *Social Research Briefs,* 11. [Online]. Available: nchsr.arts.unsw.edu.au/media/File/SRB11.pdf [Accessed 25 July 2011].

Poynard T (2002). *Hepatitis B and C: management and treatment.* London: Martin Dunitz.

Verdoux H. (2004) Cannabis and psychosis proneness. In D Castle & R Murray (Eds). *Marijuana and madness: psychiatry and neurobiology* (pp75–88). New York: Cambridge University Press.

Zickmund S, Bryce C, Blasiole J, Shinkunas L, LaBrecque D & Arnold R (2006). Majority of patients with hepatitis C express physical, mental and social difficulties with antiviral treatment. *European Journal of Gastroenterology and Hepatology*, 18: 381–88.

Chapter 6

Applying data mining to a cohort of acute traumatic brain injury admissions: our experiences

Glade Vyslysel and Lisa Channon

This chapter reports the findings of a clinical data-mining project which explored the patient journey of those admitted to an acute hospital with traumatic brain injury (TBI). The study focused on post-traumatic amnesia testing, occupational therapy input and discharge planning. Clinical guidelines recommend that acute patients admitted with TBI have early referral to occupational therapy and are assessed with the Westmead Post Traumatic Amnesia Scale (WPTAS). Concern about the efficacy of our occupational therapy department's management of this patient population motivated the authors to undertake this initiative.

The study audited the records of 311 TBI admissions over a 12-month period. It found that over half of admissions were aged between 16 and 35 years, nearly 60% of all admissions resulted from a motor vehicle accident and that 94% received assessment and intervention. This study identified a gap in recommended service delivery relating to the provision of patient education. This chapter documents evidence that, with some academic support and despite time and resource constraints, full-time clinicians can successfully mine routinely collected data, analyse service delivery, identify evidence–practice gaps and potentially improve the healthcare provided to patients admitted to an acute hospital setting.

Key words: data mining, traumatic brain injury, post-traumatic amnesia testing, occupational therapy

Traumatic brain injury (TBI) is a non-degenerative, non-congenital insult to the brain from an external mechanical force such as a fall, motor vehicle accident or assault. It can result in temporary or permanent impairment of cognitive, physical, and psychosocial functions (Dawodu 2009). Recovery and outcomes are not only affected by the severity of the injury, but also by pre-injury factors such as personality, coping mechanisms, and social and environmental supports (Reed 2007).

TBI is one of the leading causes of death and disability worldwide (Bruns & Hauser 2003). Most statistical reports quantifying management of TBI in acute hospitals are based on the International Classification of Disease (ICD) codes. These codes offer a standard diagnostic classification of 'the incidence and prevalence of diseases and other health problems in relation to variables such as the characteristics and circumstances of the individuals affected, reimbursement and resource allocation' (World Health Organization 2010). National 2004 and 2005 ICD data analysed by the Australian Institute of Health and Welfare (Helps et al. 2008) revealed that there were 22,710 individuals hospitalised with TBI, with the estimated costs of $184 million dollars. TBI affects all age groups; however, 63% of individuals injured are of working age between 16 to 64 years (Motor Accident Authority 2008).

TBI is often classified as mild, moderate or severe according to the severity of the initial injury (Rimmel et al. 1981). The Glasgow Coma Scale (GCS) is an ordinal scale that is often used to measure the severity of injury (Teasdale & Jennett 1974). A score of 13 to 15 indicates mild brain injury, 9 to 12 a moderate injury, and 3 to 8 a severe brain injury. According to the World Health Organization, mild TBI comprises 70–90% of all adult hospital TBI admission (Cassidy et al. 2004), moderate injuries account for approximately 10% of admissions, and severe injuries a further 10%.

Post-traumatic amnesia is another TBI outcome often used to measure the severity of brain injury (Ponsford et al. 2004). It is considered by the New South Wales Institute of Trauma and Injury Management (Reed 2007) as the best predictor of the development of post-concussive syndrome. Post-traumatic amnesia is defined by

Levin, O'Donnell and Grossman (1979, p675) as 'an interval during which the patient is confused, amnesic for ongoing events and likely to evidence behavioural disturbance'. The Westmead Post Traumatic Amnesia Scale (WPTAS) (Marosszeky et al. 1997) is an assessment used to measure post-traumatic amnesia. A mild injury is sustained if a person is assessed as amnesic for less than a day; a moderate injury if amnesia lasts between one and seven days and a severe injury if greater than seven days. The importance of accurately assessing the length of amnesia is very important as it is considered, in conjunction with the GCS, to be the 'gold standard' assessment for measuring injury severity. The WPTAS is a good predictor of cognitive recovery and functional outcome, and important to medico-legal practice (Khan et al. 2003; Tate et al. 2005).

Post-concussive syndrome can arise as a result of cerebral dysfunction or the psychological consequences of TBI (Wiley & Strauman 2000). Post-concussive symptoms, as noted by Sheedy et al. (2009), can include somatic complaints such as headache, dizziness and nausea, cognitive deficits (including poor concentration and memory) and affective problems such as depression, frustration and irritability. According to the Diagnostic and Statistical Manual of Mental Disorders (American Psychiatric Association 1994), a post-concussive disorder is a clinical state in which head trauma is accompanied by three or more post-concussive symptoms persisting for greater than three months after an injury. Research suggests that the early diagnosis of mild TBI and education of post-concussive symptoms helps to avoid the development of chronic post-TBI sequel (Borg et al. 2004). In New South Wales, Australia, clinical guidelines recommend early referral and management for all TBI patients, the completion of post-traumatic amnesia testing using the WPTAS and the provision of education on TBI recovery (Motor Accident Authority 2008; Reed 2007).

In recent years, there has been increasing demand to provide statistical evidence of the impact of changes in clinical practice. This growth has led to a review of the quality of the data currently recorded by clinicians within the Occupational Therapy Department at John Hunter Hospital. The accessibility of relevant data sources has assisted us in demonstrating the achievements being made as well as the department's commitment to quality improvement.

While it is well recognised that the demand for access to quality healthcare is continuing to increase (O'Connell et al. 2008), it is also understood that 'the available budget will always be less than the potential service delivery options,' (Hunter New England Area Health Service 2008, p8). As such, it is essential that clinicians are able to utilise cost effective and reliable data sources that they can both contribute to and draw upon time-efficient and sustainable formats.

Following involvement in data-mining workshops initiated by the HNE Allied Health Research Committee and facilitated by Professor Epstein, it was determined that an existing statistical program, the Allied Health Management Information System (AHMIS), was a potentially useful source for our occupational therapy department. A number of early quality projects were implemented to ensure therapists consistently entered statistical information into AHMIS that included brightly coloured 'cheat sheets' located on all computers, regular focus groups and random spot checks of therapists' coding accuracy. These strategies improved coding consistency and enabled us to use AHMIS as a data source for our TBI post-traumatic amnesia testing data-mining project.

At John Hunter Hospital all post-traumatic amnesia testing is completed by occupational therapists. Two standardised measures, the Westmead Post Traumatic Amnesia Scale (WPTAS) (Marosszeky et al. 1997; Reed 2007) and the Abbreviated Westmead Post Traumatic Amnesia Scale (Motor Accident Authority 2008; Shores et al. 2008), are used to complete this testing. In this paper, both scales will be referred to collectively as the WPTA scale.

Our clinical experience indicated that the TBI population was a resource-intensive clinical group. Therapists working across a range of clinical specialties (for example, neurosurgery or orthopaedics) were responsible for completing the WPTA scale. They commonly reported a number of concerns about the utilisation of assessment and management of this clinical group. These concerns included an uncertainty as to the quantity of TBI admissions to the hospital, the number of missing or delayed referrals to occupational therapy, inadequate discharge timeframes, and concern about clinicians' ability to not only assess, but to also achieve therapy goals and provide patient and family education. To investigate these concerns a retrospective cohort study was undertaken. However, this chapter is not just a report of study outcomes, but also a reflection on our experiences as clinicians undertaking a practice-driven research initiative which mined existing clinical data.

Aims of the study

The authors were interested in exploring the rates, demography and patient 'journey' of working age TBI admissions, the current utilisation of the WPTAS and the provision of TBI patient education. This study will describe:

- the demography of TBI admissions
- the patients' acute hospital journey, including the admitting speciality and ward location
- how many TBI patients received the WPTA assessment
- occupational therapy referral patterns and the amount of face-to-face contact time
- the frequency and type of occupational therapy interventions provided
- the reflective journey of the authors during this data-mining project.

Methodology

Organisational context

The John Hunter Hospital is a 550-bed tertiary referral hospital and is the only trauma centre outside of Sydney, the capital city of New South Wales. Its occupational therapy department uses an evidence-based, client-centred approach to optimise function post-injury and/or illness. Therapists manage patients admitted with TBI using the WPTAS. All TBI interventions are aimed at enabling participation in everyday activities. The overarching goal of the occupational therapist in an acute setting is to facilitate safe and appropriate hospital discharge.

Sample

The study audited the records of all patients diagnosed with TBI, admitted between 1 April 2009 and 31 March 2010, aged between 16 and 65 years. Patients over the age of 65 years were excluded because the WPTAS has not been validated for adults over 65 years. For the purposes of our data-mining project, additional TBI data was collected from the hospital ICD codes relating to concussion, loss of consciousness, and post-traumatic amnesia.

Data sources and collection process

This study utilised two data sources. Firstly AHMIS, a source that is readily available to occupational therapists as part of their routine clinical work was used for data mining. Most aspects of allied health clinical and non-clinical work are recorded in the AHMIS statistical program. Therapists record a patient's therapy diagnosis, admitting medical speciality, and any patient-related interventions. For the purposes of this study, only direct face-to-face clinical time was audited. All patients presenting with TBI were entered into AHMIS using a TBI diagnosis-specific code. This data were cross-matched with the intervention code designated for administration of the WPTAS. This cross-matching ensured that any patients with cognitive problems that were not related to TBI were excluded from the study. This data source only included patients referred for occupational therapy.

Secondly, TBI admissions that had not been referred to occupational therapy for WPTAS were identified using hospital admissions with TBI-related ICD codes. Once these two datasets were combined, any additional 'missing' data were obtained using the inpatient Patient Management systems, the Digital Medical Record and/or the Clinical Access Program. This process provided a complete dataset for the 12-month period. All data was entered into a Microsoft Excel spreadsheet for tabulation and exported to Statistical Package for the Social Sciences (SPSS) for analysis. Results were analysed using a one-way ANOVA (Analysis of Variance between groups).

Results

Demography of TBI admissions and administration of the WPTA scale

This study audited 311 TBI admissions over the 12-month period (Table 6.1). Of the 311 patients, 94% were referred to occupational therapy for administration of the WPTA scale, 76% were male, with the highest frequencies clustered in equal amounts in the 16–25 and 26–35 year age brackets. The number of admissions reduced with age, with only 11.9% in the final group 56–65 years. During this 12-month period, 60% of TBI admissions resulted from a motor vehicle or motor bike accident, 13.5% from an injury including falls, and 10.9% from assault.

The acute hospital journey of TBI patients

Nearly 70% of patients were admitted under general surgical or neurosurgical specialities with only 18.9% admitted under orthopaedics (Table 6.1). Two-thirds of all admissions were managed on wards specifically designated for patients under these specialities. However, 16% of patients were managed in an emergency short-stay ward and a further 16% were admitted as 'outliers'.

In terms of discharge destination, a total of two-thirds of all patients were discharged home from the acute hospital setting, and 12.5% of this group required the support of family. A further 14.5% were transferred to a rehabilitation facility, while 7.4% were transferred to another acute hospital.

Occupational therapy referral patterns

Only 5.5% (n=17) of TBI admissions were not referred to occupational therapy for administration of the WPTA scale. More than 50% of these were discharged from the emergency short stay ward. The mean time between admission and referral was 3.6 days (SD = 12.0); however, there was a large degree of variability between patients, which is reflected in Figure 6.1. A one-way ANOVA test was applied to identify if the time between admission and referral was different across medical specialties. It showed that there was no significant difference (p = .911).

Table 6.1: Demographic and acute hospital journey information

Data item	Descriptors	Frequency	Percentage
Number of admissions	March 2009–April 2010	311	100
Occupational therapy referral received	Yes	294	94.5
	No	17	5.5
Gender	Male	237	76.2
	Female	74	23.8
Age	16–25 years	81	26
	26–35 years	82	26.4
	36–45 years	64	20.6
	46–55 years	47	15.1
	56–65 years	37	11.9
Mechanism of injury	Transport	185	59.5
	Fall	42	13.5
	Assault	34	10.9
	Cyclist	13	4.2
	Other	24	7.7
	Unknown	13	4.2
Admitting speciality	Surgery	115	36.9
	Neurosurgery	99	31.7
	Orthopaedics	59	18.9
	Emergency Medicine	22	7.1
	Otolaryngology Maxillofacial	12	3.9
	Other Medicine Specialties	4	1.5

Data item	Descriptors	Frequency	Percentage
Hospital ward	Neurosurgery	74	23.8
	Orthopaedics	58	18.6
	General Surgery	45	14.5
	Special Surgery	34	10.9
	Emergency Short Stay	50	16.1
	Other	50	16.1
Discharge destination	Home	169	54.3
	Home with Supervision or Relatives/Friends' Home	39	12.5
	Rehab Facility	45	14.5
	T/F Another Acute Facility	23	7.4
	Remains an Inpatient	9	2.9
	Unknown	27	8.4

Note. T/F = transfer

Figure 6.1: Comparison of time between admission and referral

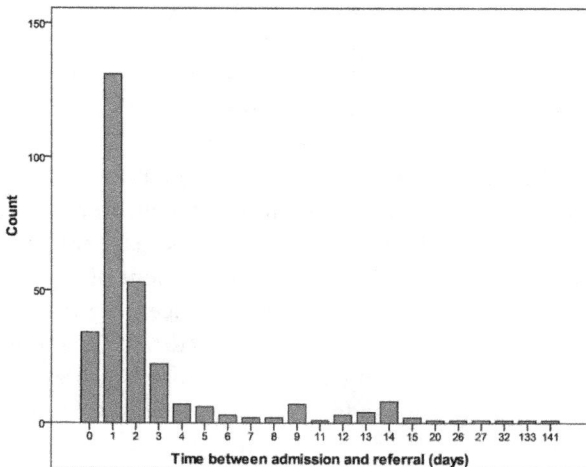

Table 6.2: Occupational therapy interventions and outcomes

Data Item	Outcome information	Frequency	Percentage
Occupational therapy	WPTAS	294	94.5
Top three additional interventions	Education on health maintenance and recovery	80	27.2
	Assessment of health maintenance and recovery	34	11.5
	Assessment of situation, occupation and environment	19	6.4
Outcome of intervention	Goals achieved	111	37.7
	Goals partly achieved	99	33.7
	Discharge therapy incomplete	51	17.3
	Discharge assessment only	6	2.0
	Self discharge	4	2.0
	Unknown	23	7.8

Note. WPTAS = Westmead Post Traumatic Amnesia Scale

Occupational therapy direct contact time and interventions

On average, patients received 72 minutes (range 10–975) of total 'face to face' time with an occupational therapist, across an average of four (range 1–48) occasions of service (OOS). In total, 1185 occasions of service were provided for TBI-related admissions; with 22.5% of patients receiving ≥ 5 and 24.4% receiving ≤ 1. A total of 139 patients (44.7%) received additional occupational therapy interventions. Of the 24 additional interventions provided, the most frequent were education on health maintenance and recovery (27.2%), the assessment of health maintenance and recovery (11.5%) and assessment of a patient's situation, occupation or environment (6.4%). Concerning the completion of intervention on discharge, results indicated that 71.4% of patients were discharged with goals fully (n = 111) or partly achieved (n = 99). Therapy remained incomplete for 17.3% of patients. Of the remaining patients, only 2.0% had been seen by an occupational therapist at the time of discharge and 2.0% self-discharged. The outcome of the remaining 7.8% of patients seen by occupational therapy remains unknown.

Discussion

Undertaking research as practicing clinicians can be challenging. Throughout our data-mining project we experienced a number of hurdles which included departmental and financial restraints and the inability to source additional funding for statistical analysis in a timely manner. We also faced the daily challenge of trying to balance the demands of busy clinical case loads with the time-intensive process of reviewing literature and processing data. In addition we had a number of staff changes within our department which impacted on our time and our ability to prioritise progress and complete our project.

Between us, we had limited experience conducting data-mining projects on this scale. As our project progressed we realised that we were lacking clarity about the direction of our investigation. It became very clear to us that as practising clinicians we would really benefit from mentoring and support from more experienced researchers to help us to define and focus our ideas to a more manageable volume. We were fortunate that in our facility we already had working relationships with some researchers that we were able to approach to support us with our data-mining project. We would encourage all future clinicians wanting to be involved in data mining to set up mentoring and supervision early in their projects.

As inexperienced researchers, we grossly underestimated the time required to obtain a complete dataset. Our early work matching ICD codes and AHMIS highlighted a number of discrepancies and missing data. In a number of cases we needed to manually check patients' medical discharge summaries and admission information to confirm a diagnosis of TBI, ward location and length of stay (LOS). It was fortuitous that our hospital had recently adopted a Digital Medical Record program and this and the other relevant data sources could be accessed from our own offices through intranet systems.

Interestingly, up to 39% of all patients within the occupational therapy AHMIS dataset coded as having TBI and requiring a WPTAS assessment were not recorded in the hospital ICD codes under the three diagnostic codes of post-traumatic amnesia, loss of consciousness or concussion. This raised a number of more broad concerns for us related to the collection of national data based exclusively on hospital ICD codes (Helps et al. 2008). It is possible that this method of data collection underestimates the frequency of TBI admissions. Inaccuracy of ICD codes may have a number of implications including inadequately quantifying the number of people sustaining TBI, difficulties predicting the resourcing required for this group in addition to increased difficulties identifying areas of priority for injury prevention.

Despite these challenges, this data-mining project has proven to be a very valuable exercise for our occupational therapy department. It enabled us to connect the compulsory daily grind of statistical entry to clinical questions and answers of relevance to our department. We are hopeful that this increased meaningful outcome from the data entry process has not only improved accuracy but increased our confidence in understanding its nature, quality and impact of our daily work. As our data-mining project progressed, we realised that we should have included more data relating to the administrative and indirect patient activities that we spend with this clinical group. Our data indicated that we spent on average 72 minutes with patients, but that did not include any time spent writing in medical records, preparing resources and consulting with others. We would encourage other future data miners to include non-clinical time that contributes to providing effective patient care.

The data-mining project also highlighted some areas for service improvement. In the 12-month study period, only 27.2% of patients had statistical data entered for the provision of TBI recovery education. The clinical guidelines report that all patients admitted with TBI should have not only access to WPTAS assessment but also the appropriate TBI education (Motor Accidents Authority 2008). It is possible that some broader hospital processes may impact on the ability of the occupational therapist to routinely provide this education, including the transfer of patients to other facilities (22%). In these instances it would be standard practice for occupational therapists to hand over the care and ongoing interventions to colleagues in the receiving facility, although it was beyond the scope of our project to identify if this did or didn't happen. There are other possible factors influencing an occupational therapist's ability to provide education including discharges by medical team prior to the completion of occupational therapy, self discharge or missing referrals (32.1%).

The results of our data-mining project also identified some discrepancies in occupational therapy input related to a patient's location within the hospital. Of the relatively small numbers of patients not referred to occupational therapy, 50% of these were located on an emergency short stay unit. Short stay units have been designed to provide a short period of assessment for patient groups who no longer require emergency department care. Effective implementation of short stay units requires a proactive team of dedicated nurses, medical staff and referral access to allied health staff including occupational therapists (NSW Health 2010). The findings of our study will assist the occupational therapy department to better target the provision of education for short-stay patients admitted with TBI, ensuring that both nursing and medical residents and registrars, who frequently rotate through specialties in teaching hospitals such as this one, are familiar with the referral, assessment and management process for people admitted with TBI.

Limitations

A number of factors may influence the interpretation of our results. Firstly, it was difficult to ensure high consistency of data coding and entry across multiple therapists. Even though we had completed a number of early quality projects that focused on coding accuracy, we were surprised that only 27.2% of patients were coded as having received education on TBI recovery. Anecdotally, all therapists within our department reported that they routinely provided this education and therefore may not have been separating it out statistically from providing a WPTAS assessment. Secondly, non-face-to-face clinical time was not included in our data collection phase. This omission may have underestimated the true clinical resources required to service this population.

Further data mining regarding a patient's journey through the hospital may have provided us with more information about influences on referral times for example, had a patient been in intensive care prior to referral. This could have been combined with information on the admission Glasgow Coma Scale (GCS) to give further information on the severity of the TBI and the incidences of mild, moderate and severe TBI. This information may also have assisted us to separate the WPTAS assessment into the 'standard' WPTAS and the 'abbreviated' WPTAS so that we could identify whether or not we were applying these assessment in a way that met the relevant clinical guidelines.

Conclusion

Our data-mining project has given us greater insight into the frequency, intensity and resource requirements of people admitted with TBI who require the WPTAS assessment in our hospital. The overall outcome of this data-mining project suggests that occupational therapists at our hospital are managing TBI patients with reasonable success both in terms of the referral of patients for assessment (94%) and full or partial achievement of patient goals on discharge (71.4%). However, we are now more aware of areas where further multidisciplinary staff education is required in order that all TBI patients receive nationally recommended assessment, education and care.

This data-mining project provides an example of how full-time clinicians with adequate access to appropriate mentoring and support can overcome everyday barriers and effectively utilise existing data sources to complete data-mining initiatives. This project has not only given us an increased understanding of the pathways of care for people admitted with TBI into this acute setting, but it has also increased our confidence to utilise existing clinical data sources to identify our current clinical practice, to reveal evidence–practice gaps and, in turn, to direct future service delivery improvements.

Acknowledgments

We would like to acknowledge the support of Ms Isobel Hubbard who helped us in the writing and editing of this chapter, and Dr Anne Vertigan who helped us with the statistical analysis. We would also like to acknowledge our occupational therapy manager Mary-Anne Barlas, our colleague Janet Frith who helped with early quality projects, our occupational therapy assistant Eden Maher and all the occupational therapists who continue to faithfully enter the AHMIS data and to respond to TBI referrals.

References

American Psychiatric Association (1994). *Diagnostic and statistical manual of mental disorders*. 4th edn. Washington DC: American Psychiatric Association.

Borg J, Holm L, Cassidy JD, Peloso PM, Carroll LJ, van Holst H & Ericson K (2004). Diagnostic procedures in mild traumatic brain injury: results of the WHO collaborating centre task force on mild traumatic brain injury. *Journal of Rehabilitation Medicine*, 43(supplement): 61–75.

Bruns J Jr & Hauser WA (2003). The epidemiology of traumatic brain injury: a review. *Epilepsia*, 44(s10): 2–10.

Cassidy JD, Carroll LJ, Peloso PM, Borg J, von Holst H, Holm L, Kraus J & Coronado VG (2004). Incidence, risk factors and prevention of mild traumatic brain injury: results of the WHO collaborating centre task force on mild traumatic brain injury. *Journal of Rehabilitation Medicine*, 43(supplement): 28–60.

Corrigan JD, Selassie AW & Orman JA (2010). The epidemiology of traumatic brain injury. *Journal of Head Trauma and Rehabilitation*, 25(2): 72–80.

Dawodu ST (2009). Traumatic brain injury (TBI): definition, epidemiology, pathophysiology. [Online]. Available: emedicine.medscape.com/article/326510-overview [Accessed 25 March 2011].

Helps Y, Henley G & Harrison JE (2008). *Hospital separations due to traumatic brain injury. Australia 2004–2005*. Injury Research and Statistics Series Number 45 (Cat no. INJCAT 116). Adelaide: Australian Institute of Health and Welfare.

Hunter New England Area Health Service (2008). *A new direction for Hunter New England: Health Service strategic plan towards 2010.* New Lambton: Hunter New England Area Health Service.

Khan F, Baguley IJ & Cameron ID (2003). Rehabilitation after traumatic brain injury. *The Medical Journal of Australia*, 178(6): 290–95.

Levin HS, O'Donnell VW & Grossman RG (1979). The Galveston orientation and amnesia test: a practical scale to assess cognition after head injury. *Journal of Nervous and Mental Disease*, 167: 675–84.

Marosszeky NEV, Ryan L, Shores EA, Batchelor J & Marosszeky JE (1997). *The PTA protocol: guidelines for using the Westmead Post-Traumatic Amnesia (PTA) scale.* Sydney: Wild & Wooley.

Motor Accident Authority NSW. (2008). *Guidelines for mild traumatic brain injury following closed head injury: acute/post-acute assessment and management.* Sydney: Motor Accident Authority NSW.

Murray CJL & Lopez AD (1996). *Global health statistics: a compendium of incidence, prevalence and mortality estimates for over 200 conditions.* Cambridge, MA: Harvard University Press.

New South Wales Health (2010). New models of emergency care: reference guide – short say units. [Online]. Available: www.archi.net.au/documents/e-library/models/emergency_care/short_stay/shortstay-units.pdf [Accessed 25 March 2010].

O'Connell TJ, Ben-Tovim DI, McCaughan BC, Szwarcbord MG & McGrath KM (2008). Health services under siege: the case for clinical process redesign. *Medical Journal of Australia*, 188(6 supplement): S9–S11.

Ponsford J, Cameron P, Wilmott C, Rothwell A, Kelly AM, Nelms R & Ng K (2004). Use of the Westmead PTA Scale to monitor recovery of memory after mild head injury. *Brain Injury*, 18(4): 603–14.

Reed D (2007). *Adult trauma clinical practice guidelines: initial management of closed head injury in adults.* North Ryde: NSW Institute of Trauma and Injury Management.

Rimmel RW, Giordani B, Barth JT, Boll TJ & Jane JA (1981). Disability caused by minor head injury. *Neurosurgery*, 9: 221–28.

Sheedy J, Harvey E, Faux S, Geffen G & Shores EA (2009). Emergency department assessment of mild traumatic brain injury and the prediction of post concussive symptoms: a three-month prospective study. *Journal of Head Trauma Rehabilitation*, 24(5): 333–43.

Shores EA, Lammél A, Hullick C, Sheedy J, Flynn M, Levick W & Batchelor J (2008). The diagnostic accuracy of the Revised Westmead PTA Scale as an adjunct to the Glasgow Coma Scale in the early identification of cognitive impairment in patients with mild traumatic brain injury. *Journal of Neurology, Neurosurgery and Psychiatry*, 79: 1100–06.

Tate RL, Pfaff A, Hodgkinsons AE, Baruley IJ, Guka JA, Marosszeky JE & King C (2004). Post-traumatic amnesia: an investigation into the validity of measuring instruments. Final report to funding body: Motor Accidents Authority of New South Wales. [Online]. Available: www.lifetimecare.nsw.gov.au/Brain_Injury.aspx [Accessed 12 May 2010].

Teasdale G & Jennett B (1974). Assessment of coma and impaired consciousness: a practical scale. *Lancet*, 2: 81–84.

Wiley M & Strauman S (2000). Diagnosis of mild head injury and the post concussion syndrome. *Journal of Head Trauma Rehabilitation*, 15(2): 783–91.

World Health Organization. (2010). International Classification of Diseases (ICD). [Online]. Available: www.who.int/classifications/icd/en/ [Accessed 29 November 2010].

Chapter 7

Treating lost language: speech pathology management of aphasia in the acute hospital setting

Luisa Renna and Anne E Vertigan

Losing the ability to communicate verbally or understand spoken words and conversation can have devastating psycho-social consequences. For some patients admitted to hospital with stroke and other brain injury this loss of language can be a profound, life-changing occurrence. Aphasia refers to a language impairment resulting from brain injury. Speech pathology assessment and treatment for speech and language deficits following brain injury forms an integral part of clinical management within the acute hospital phase for patients with stroke. This clinical data-mining project evolved following the implementation of a formal standardised aphasia test in the acute hospital setting, the Bedside Evaluation Screening Test for Aphasia – 2 (BEST-2), applicable to such patients. Despite growing evidence regarding the benefits of providing early and high frequency aphasia therapy, aphasia therapy is typically a lower priority in the acute setting, with dysphagia (swallowing) management often consuming the majority of speech pathology time. This clinical data-mining project provides a profile of aphasia assessment and therapy in the acute setting and discusses future directions and speech pathology service delivery within this population.

Key words: aphasia, language disorder, aphasia therapy, stroke

Aphasia is a language impairment caused by damage to the language centres of the brain following stroke or other brain injury (Chapey 1986). Aphasia has devastating consequences for the individual and their family and can lead to frustration, embarrassment, depression and loss of autonomy about their medical care as well as daily living. Aphasia can be multi-modal across communication domains affecting writing, reading, speaking and listening (Davis 2000).

Stroke is now Australia's leading cause of disability, with 67% of acute patients presenting with communication deficits (National Stroke Foundation 2009). Studies have demonstrated that as many as 38% of patients admitted to acute hospitals with stroke will have aphasia (Bakheit et al. 2007; Engelter et al. 2006.). In addition to aphasia, stroke and other brain injuries can also cause dysphagia (swallowing difficulties) and dysarthria by affecting the muscles required for producing clear speech (National Stroke Foundation 2009).

Despite the devastating effects that aphasia can have on patients and their families, therapy, including education and family support, is not a high priority for treatment in some acute hospital settings. Frequently, dysphagia is assessed and managed more thoroughly than communication disorders. This often stems from the knowledge that dysphagia can result in serious medical complications and can be life threatening in some cases (McCooey-O'Halloran et al. 2004). Studies have demonstrated an increase in dysphagia referrals to speech pathology in Australian acute hospital settings concurrently, along with increased aphasia referrals (Enderby & Petheram 2002; Armstrong 2003). Typically, however, there is no increase in speech pathology resources to coincide with these increased referrals.

Since emphasis is commonly placed on dysphagia, there is limited information about current practice in aphasia assessment and therapy within acute hospital settings. In order to establish best practice for aphasia therapy in this primary treatment venue, it is important to understand the profile of patients presenting with aphasia. The purpose of this study is to analyse formal language assessment data from patients post-brain injury and to outline the therapy provided to these patients using a clinical data-mining approach (Epstein 2010). More specifically, this paper uses available clinical data to profile patients admitted to acute hospitals with aphasia post-brain injury, in particular stroke, and to study speech pathology interventions provided to this subgroup. It also seeks to determine the influence of patient demographics, handedness and stroke classification on assessment results.

Literature review

Traditionally patients with stroke or brain injury in the acute phase of hospitalisation have been deemed unsuitable for impairment-based aphasia therapy due to the impact of spontaneous recovery (Holland & Fridrikkson 2001), the fear of medical complications, and ward environments that are not conducive to therapy (Lalor & Cranfield 2004). Therefore a common assumption is that impairment-based therapy is unsuitable in the acute phase. Such theories have also been supported by conflicting levels of evidence both promoting and refuting the benefits of acute aphasia therapy, as shown by Greener et al's systematic Cochrane review (2000) where acute aphasia therapy was neither shown to be clearly effective nor clearly ineffective.

Consequently, the argument *for* aphasia therapy during acute care remains controversial. In a literature review, Holland and Fridrikkson (2001) reported that patients benefit more from supportive conversational and education-based therapy during the acute phase compared to more impairment-based therapies. Their controlled clinical trial found that conversational–counselling therapy, which includes emotional support, conversational activities and aphasia education, was more effective than impairment-based therapy such as structured divergent naming tasks combined with conversational language treatment. However Peach (2001) subsequently claimed that there is a lack of strong scientific evidence to support the findings of Holland and Fridrikkson. Peach pointed out that Holland and Fridrikkson's study did not account for changes in stroke severity, was comprised of a small sample and that at one month post-assessment no difference in language deficits between the two intervention groups remained. All authors agreed, however, that further research was required before definite claims could be made about the utility of aphasia therapy in the acute setting.

More recently, similar questions have been raised by Bhogal, Teasell, Speechley and Albert (2003). In their systematic analysis of aphasia therapy in acute care, significantly shorter periods but more intensive hours of therapy resulted in improved language skills compared to longer sessions with less frequent therapy. This conclusion is confirmed within a recent Cochrane review (Brady & Enderby 2010) where intensive therapy was found to be more effective than conventional therapy. In accordance with these results a recent Australian randomised control trial (RCT) study, presented at the 2008 Stroke Society of Australasia conference (Godecke et al. 2008), demonstrated significantly improved communication effectiveness for patients with moderate to severe aphasia at acute hospital discharge and six months later with daily aphasia therapy versus weekly aphasia therapy in hospital. A current, rigorously designed RCT by Laska et al. (2008) is investigating the efficacy of aphasia therapy in the acute phase, and should provide more solid empirical evidence to inform decision-making about aphasia therapy in the acute phase.

Equally promising is the fact that stroke rehabilitation research is currently investigating brain neuroplasticity and the effects of enriching treatment environments for patients with stroke and brain injury. Burns (2008) discusses such advances and the potential benefits of applying neuroplasticity research and principles to aphasia therapy in stroke populations. These principles include high-intensity repetitive practice, attention tasks and cross-training of cognitive skills to enhance therapeutic efficacy and efficiency.

But stroke and brain injury patients continue to be admitted to hospital while we wait for conclusive evidence. At this moment in time, it is both theoretically and practically plausible to consider that early and intense aphasia intervention could be beneficial to promote language recovery.

In light of new research suggesting that more intensive aphasia therapy might be effective in the context of acute care, current speech pathology service delivery in Australian acute hospitals is of interest. Accordingly, Armstrong (2003) and McCooey-O'Halloran et al. (2004) discuss recent changes to speech pathology service delivery in Australian hospitals, especially in regards to the prioritisation of dysphagia over acute speech and language disorders. Both papers raise concerns not only for the maintenance of speech pathology skills in acquired speech and language disorders within the acute setting, but also for the knowledge and awareness of the professional speech pathologist's role within the multidisciplinary team. Such concerns are discussed by Lalor and Cranfield (2004) in a descriptive study conducted within an Australian acute hospital service. Over a 12-month period, 40 out of 59 patients formally identified as aphasic received no communication therapy because of large speech pathology caseload demands. Of the 59, 32 were treated for dysphagia only, while a total of 13 received aphasia therapy. This is one of the first studies to investigate both the incidence of aphasia, its epidemiology and to consider the suitability of patients for aphasia therapy.

Proper implementation of aphasia therapy requires sound, differential assessment. A number of factors affecting aphasia assessment in the acute hospital setting include changes in neurological status and unanticipated medical setbacks as well as factors in the ward environments (Holland et al. 2001). For example, patients in the acute phase may experience rapid neurological deterioration or spontaneous recovery, rendering prior formal testing results invalid. Alternatively, ward environments can be noisy and unregulated, causing frequent interruptions to assessment and treatment protocols. Although extensive diagnostic testing may not be appropriate, the promotion of formal ward-based assessment protocols can be beneficial for ensuring inter-clinician reliability and comprehensive analysis of language deficits (Peach 2001). Fortunately, many formal aphasia screening assessments have been shown to have strong inter-reliability and can be administered in a short period, offsetting acute hospital constraints. Most are also reproducible, making possible changes in language function measurement on a daily or weekly basis. For example, the Bedside Evaluation Screening Test for Aphasia (BEST-2) (West et al. 1988) is a standardised language assessment tool designed for use in the acute setting to provide information on specific language deficits, allowing individual subtest and total severity scores. Patients are given an overall impairment rating which is classified as either (a) severe, (b) moderate, or (c) mild to within normal limits (WNL). The *mild* and *within normal limits* severity categories are grouped together. Therefore differentiation between the *mild* and *within normal limits* categories cannot be determined within this test.

The BEST-2 can be useful in profiling aphasia in the acute hospital setting and identifying specific language deficits in a formalised manner. It contains a number of subtests which are described in Table 7.1. Designed to be administered in the acute setting, it is short and adaptable and provides additional information on language deficits and responses to levels of cueing and stimulation (West et al. 1988). It is, however, a screening assessment tool and does not eradicate the need for *in-depth* language assessment with some patients. Patients presenting with more high-level language aphasia or cognitive communication disorders may not be identified easily on the BEST-2, and hence may fall within the mild-WNL subgroup. Still, such patients will often present with language deficits in conversational and more complex language tasks during assessment.

Table 7.1: Description of BEST-2 subtest tasks

Subtest	Description
Conversational expression	Conversational expression from directed questions
Object naming	Verbal naming of objects
Describing objects	Verbal description of objects
Repeating	Sentence repetition following a verbal model
Pointing to objects	Identification of objects in response to auditory command
Pointing to parts of a picture	Identification of parts of a picture from an auditory command
Reading	Comprehending written words, sentences and paragraphs

Aphasia assessment information also needs to be interpreted in the context of patient demographics, handedness and stroke classification. Handedness can provide important clues to a patient's laterality of motor functions within the brain (Davies 2000). Evidence suggests that right-handed people represent language on the left side of the brain whereas left-handed people may have a more bilateral representation (Davies, 2000). It is therefore important to identify handedness when interpreting results of aphasia assessment. The Oxfordshire stroke classification system (Bamford et al. 1990) is a well-researched classification model which is used for the classification of stroke sub-type at the bedside. This classification is used in conjunction with other tests, such as brain imaging, to provide important information on stroke severity and prognosis and is a tool recommended by the Australian National Stroke Foundation (National Stroke Foundation 2009). Stroke is classified as either (1) Total Anterior Circulation Stroke (TAC), (2) Partial Anterior Circulation Stroke (PAC), (3) Lacunar Stroke (LAC), or (4) Posterior Circulation Stroke (POC). This classification allows judgements to be made on location of stroke within the brain and concurrent deficits that are likely to exist (see Table 7.2).

Organisational context

The Greater Newcastle Acute Hospital Network Speech Pathology Department is located at John Hunter Hospital (JHH) and Belmont District Hospital (BDH) in Newcastle. JHH is the principal referral centre, teaching hospital and community hospital for Newcastle and is the only trauma centre in NSW outside Sydney. John Hunter is the region's largest hospital with approximately 550 beds. Belmont Hospital is a 75-bed acute facility providing general medicine and surgery, day surgery, coronary care unit, gynaecology, neonatal, obstetrics and a 24-hour emergency department. It also contains a sub-acute four-bed stroke rehabilitation ward.

Table 7.2: Summary of the Oxfordshire classification scale (Bamford et al. 1990).

Stroke classification	Inclusive features
Total Anterior Circulation (TAC)	A combination of:
	New, higher cerebral dysfunction (dysphasia)
	Homonymous visual field defect
	Ipsilateral motor and/or sensory deficit of at least two areas out of face, arm and leg
	*If drowsy with unilateral weakness the last two factors are assumed
Partial Anterior Circulation (PAC)	No drowsiness
	2 of 3 criteria of TAC
	OR
	Higher cerebral dysfunction alone (dysphasia)
Lacunar (LAC)	Pure motor (most common)
	Sensory motor stroke
	Pure sensory stroke
	Ataxic hemiparesis
	Dysarthria, clumsy hand syndrome
Posterior Circulation (POC)	Any of:
	Brainstem, cerebellar or occipital lobe stroke
	Ipsilateral cranial nerve palsy with controlateral motor and/or sensory deficit
	Bilateral motor and/or sensory deficit
	Disorder of conjugate eye movement
	Cerebellar dysfunction without ipsilateral long tract signs
	Isolated homonymous visual field defect

Sample

For the purposes of this study, the BEST-2 was administered to all patients referred to speech pathology between February 2008 and March 2009 who had suffered a stroke or head injury (n = 100). Inclusion criteria included ability to consistently follow simple one-step commands, answer simple yes/no biographical questions, and consent to the assessment procedure. This determination was made by the assessing speech pathologist during their initial consultation. Patients were excluded if they did not meet these criteria. All participating patients were managed according to both the speech pathology department protocols, and the patient's individual needs, as determined by their treating speech pathologist. Here it is important to point out that within JHH and BDH speech pathology there is no policy that automatically prioritises dysphagia management over management of communication disorders.

Aims of the study

This study aimed to:
1. Characterise aphasia in terms of severity and deficit within the acute hospital setting using the BEST-2.
2. Explore the relationship between stroke classification and aphasia deficits and influencing factors.
3. Determine the amount and type of therapy provided to patients with aphasia in the acute and sub-acute setting.
4. Infer whether results and severity from formal language screening influenced the type and amount of therapy given.

Data sources and collection process

The BEST-2 was administered to all surviving patients by qualified speech pathologists. After 'mining' and collating all BEST-2 assessment forms, data regarding aphasia therapy provision and additional speech pathology contacts, such as dysphagia or other communication assessment and therapy, was obtained via retrospective chart review. Data regarding stroke classification, clinical syndrome, handedness and bio-graphical details were also collected.

All data were entered onto an Excel spreadsheet and exported to the Statistical Package for the Social Sciences (SPSS) version 18.0 for analysis. Language deficit, type and amount of aphasia therapy administered, age, gender, Oxfordshire stroke classification (Bamford et al. 1990), handedness and severity were analysed using descriptive statistics and one-way ANOVA.

Results

Assessment using BEST-2

Data for 100 patients (56 female, 44 male), admitted to JHH (58) and BDH (42) were available. The average age was 73 years (SD = 13, range = 37–97). The majority of patients presented with stroke (n = 90) while ten patients presented due to other neurological conditions such as Sub Arachnoid Haemorrhage (SAH) and brain tumour (Table 7.3).

Full analysis of stroke classification and handedness was not possible due to incomplete data in the medical files. Handedness was recorded in only 70 patients and of those 90% were right handed. Stroke classification using the Oxfordshire system was recorded for 52 patients. Of those classified, 83% had Total or Partial Anterior Circulation Stroke (TAC or PAC) (Table 7.3).

The average total BEST-2 severity score was 97 (SD = 16) and average total subtest score was 10 (SD = 2.5). These scores correlate to a moderate impairment level. Thirty-five patients had total scores falling in the *mild-within normal limits* (WNL) category while 23 had scores within the *severe* category.

Overall individual subtest scores were similar in average severity. Verbal naming and pointing to objects by verbal command were slightly more impaired in comparison to other subtests (Table 7.4). This finding indicated that confrontational naming of objects and following spoken commands on average proved a more difficult language task. When comparing subtest score results via severity, patients with severe deficits had more difficulty with verbal repetition and pointing to parts of a picture to a verbal command (Table 7.5). For the moderate severity group, object naming and pointing to objects by a verbal command were the most difficult subtests whereas for the mild-WNL group verbal repetition and verbal description of objects proved more difficult.

Table 7.3: Patient demographics and characteristics (n = 100)

Characteristic	Number
Medical diagnosis	
Stroke (infarct)	78
Stroke (haemorrhage)	12
Brain Tumour	4
Seizures	1
SAH/SDH	4
Aneurysm	1
Handedness	
Right	63
Left	7
Unaccounted	30
Clinical syndrome (Oxfordshire)	
TAC	21
PAC	22
LAC	4
POC	5
Other	10
Unaccounted	48

Note. TAC = Total Anterior Circulation, PAC = Partial Anterior Circulation, LAC = Lacunar Circulation, POC = Posterior Circulation, SAH = Sub Arachnoid Haemorrhage, SDH = Sub Dural Haemorrhage.

Subtest scores according to Oxfordshire classification were analysed using a one-way ANOVA (Table 7.6). There was a significant difference between groups when comparing total and individual BEST-2 subtest scores. Post hoc analysis using a Tukey test found that total score and individual subtest scores in the TAC group were significantly lower than those in the LAC (p = .016) group. There was no significant difference among other groups. Likewise, there was no statistically significant difference BEST-2 standard scores by age, gender or hospital setting.

Table 7.4: BEST-2 subtest scores for all patients

Subtest	Average Subtest Score M (SD)	Average Subtest Raw Score M (SD)
Conversational expression	10 (2.29)	21 (9)
Object naming	9 (2.50)	18 (10)
Describing objects	10 (2.63)	21 (9)
Repeating	10 (2.44)	23 (10)
Pointing to objects	9 (2.51)	20 (9)
Pointing to parts of a picture	10 (2.54)	21 (9)
Reading	10 (4.01)	14 (11)

Note. For average total scores: scores above 105 are classified as mild – within normal limits; scores between 85 and 105 are classified as moderate impairment and scores below 85 are classified as severe impairment. For individual subtest scores: scores above 11 are classified as mild – within normal limits, scores between seven and 11 are classified as moderate impairment and scores below seven are classified as severe impairment (West et al. 1988).

Table 7.5: BEST-2 subtest scores by overall aphasia severity

Subtest	Severe N (%)	Moderate N (%)	Mild – within normal limits (WNL) N (%)
Conversational expression	10	56	33
Object naming	12	64	23
Describing objects	8	56	35
Repeating	14	40	46
Pointing to objects	12	63	24
Pointing to parts of a picture	13	57	30
Reading	12	56	30

Note. For individual subtest scores: scores above 11 are classified as mild – within normal limits, scores between 7 and 11 are classified as moderate impairment and scores below 7 are classified as severe impairment (West et al. 1988).

Table 7.6: Total and subtest scores according to Oxfordshire classification analysed using a one-way ANOVA.

	TAC n = 22 M (SD)	PAC n = 22 M (SD)	LAC n = 4 M (SD)	POC n = 5 M (SD)	P value
Total Score	91.9 (14.6)	99.9 (17.6)	117.3 (2.2)	109.6 (5.9)	0.008*
Severity	1.9 (1.1)	1.3 (1.3)	0 (0)	0.5 (0.9)	0.006*
Conversational expression	8.2 (2.1)	9.8 (2.4)	12 (0)	11 (1.9)	0.004*
Naming	8.6 (2.3)	9.6 (2.5)	12.7 (0.5)	11.6 (1.7)	0.004*

	TAC n = 22 M (SD)	PAC n = 22 M (SD)	LAC n = 4 M (SD)	POC n = 5 M (SD)	P value
Description	9.5 (2.7)	10.8 (2.7)	13 (2)	12 (1.6)	0.040*
Repetition	8.6 (2.6)	10.2 (2.4)	11.7 (1.2)	11.2 (0.9)	0.022*
Pointing to objects	8.6 (2.6)	10 (2.6)	12.7 (1.3)	11 (1)	0.013*
Pointing to parts of a picture	9.1 (2.6)	10.5 (2.3)	12.7 (1.3)	10.1 (1.8)	0.027*
Reading	9 (2.6)	10.1 (2.8)	12.2 (0.5)	12 (1.7)	0.039*

Note.TAC = Total Anterior Circulation, PAC = Partial Anterior Circulation, LAC = Lacunar Circulation, POC = Posterior Circulation.

Therapy

Seventy-six out of 100 patients received aphasia therapy, with an average of 3.3 sessions per admission (SD = 4.1). On average, therapy was received every 2.5 days per length of stay (LOS). Impairment-based therapy targeting word finding was the most frequent form of therapy provided. Seventeen patients with aphasia did not receive aphasia therapy. Six of this subset died during the admission, five were discharged to another facility, such as rehabilitation, and two received other therapy for speech disorders such as dysarthria. Patients within the moderate aphasia category received the most therapy followed by those in the severe category. Furthermore, patients within the moderate and severe group received more occasions of service (OOS) overall compared to those in the mild–WNL group. For the severe group, aphasia therapy was received more frequently than other groups when comparing the ratio of therapy to length of stay. Length of stay overall was lower within the severe group compared to the moderate and mild–WNL groups. A small number of patients in the mild–WNL category received therapy, which might indicate that mild aphasia symptoms and/or cognitive communication deficits were present. Refer to Table 7.7 for further information on therapy results by severity.

The most common therapy conducted in the moderate and severe groups was impairment-based therapy targeting word finding, semantic input and auditory comprehension, including the use of alternative augmentative communication systems (e.g. training patients to communicate with spelling boards or via pictures). In contrast, the mild–WNL group received a larger amount of high level language therapy and functional generalisation language tasks and also had the longest average length of stay (LOS). Profiles of the type of therapy can be seen in Figure 7.1.

Table 7.7: Length of stay and occasions of service (OOS) according to aphasia severity category.

	Total Therapy Sessions	Aphasia Therapy OOS per patient M (SD)	LOS (days) M (SD)	Ratio of LOS to Aphasia Therapy OOS M (SD)	Ratio of LOS to total Speech Pathology OOS M (SD)
Severe (n = 23)	98	4.66 (4.6)	10.25 (7.0)	1.7 (1.5)	1.5 (1.2)
Moderate (n = 37)	144	4.8 (4.8)	15.2 (12.4)	3.0 (3.6)	2.4 (3.1)
Mild–WNL (n = 40)	86	2.3 (2.9)	16 (13.9)	3.0 (4.0)	2.9 (2.6)

Note. WNL = within normal limits; OOS = occasions of service; LOS = length of stay; M = mean; SD = standard deviation

Table 7.8: Length of stay and occasions of service by hospital

	Total Therapy Sessions	Aphasia Therapy OOS M (SD)	LOS in days M (SD)	Ratio of LOS to Aphasia Therapy OOS M (SD)	Ratio of LOS to Total Speech Pathology OOS M (SD)
JHH	140	2.91 (3.5)	9.62 (7.1)	2.0 (3.3)	2.0 (2.0)
BDH	192	4.46 (4.6)	19.79 (13.8)	3.88 (3.8)	2.93 (2.0)

Note. JHH = John Hunter Hospital; BDH = Belmont District Hospital; OOS = occasions of service; LOS = length of stay; M = mean; SD = standard deviation

Figure 7.1: Number of individual therapy interventions for 100 patients admitted during February 2008 and March 2009.

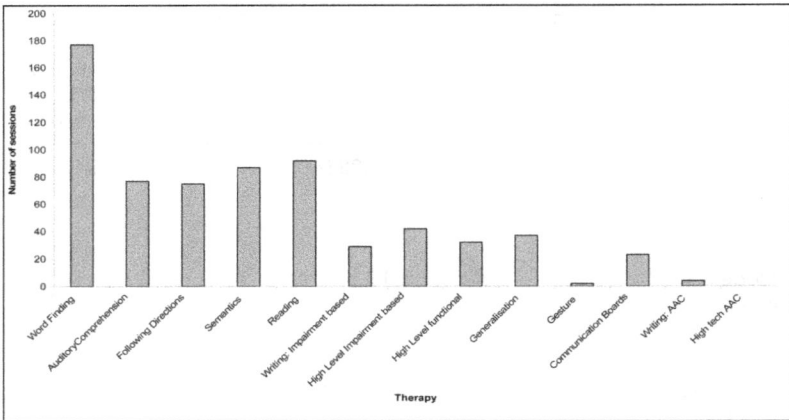

Note. Some patients received more than one type of therapy.

Discussion

This clinical data-mining study provides a profile of patients presenting with aphasia in the acute hospital setting and allows quantification of speech pathology services provided. A high percentage of patients received aphasia therapy in addition to speech pathology management for other conditions such as dysphagia and/or dysarthria. A high proportion of patients referred to speech pathology post stroke and brain injury are presenting with aphasia and have deficits in a number of language functions.

Overall, performance was more impaired on confrontational naming of objects and following spoken commands. Such language deficits may have significant consequences for the patient's ability to communicate during their hospital admission. For example, simple tasks such as requesting pain medication, following verbal instructions or understanding medical information given by hospital staff becomes extremely difficult for the individual with aphasia. These deficits can impair their progress with other therapy modalities and can increase anxiety and depression for the patient and their family.

Significant statistical differences were found when comparing available Oxfordshire classification data to BEST-2 results within individual classification groups. The TAC subgroup had significantly lower individual subtest and total language score on the BEST-2 than the LAC group. These results are consistent with the criteria within the Oxfordshire classification model that TAC criteria must include a presenting feature of aphasia whereas the LAC criteria do not.

In general, the language therapy provided was consistent with the deficits found during formal testing. For example, a higher proportion of patients had deficits in the naming subtest, and impairment-based word finding therapy was the highest proportion of therapy given. Theories as to why this is the most common therapy may be attributed to word-finding difficulties often being the most frustrating and predominant deficit for patients with aphasia post-stroke (Davies 2000). Those patients identified on the BEST-2 as severe or moderately impaired received the highest amounts of therapy. Furthermore, the severe group received more impairment-based therapy targeting word finding, auditory comprehension and semantics with additional alternative augmentative communication input. A number of patients falling within the mild–WNL group continued to demonstrate mild aphasia or cognitive communication deficits and received therapy primarily targeting high-level language, reading and functional language generalisation. These deficits, although mild, can significantly impair the individual's capacity to participate in social interactions beyond simple conversations. Therefore they may have difficulties managing personal correspondence, verbally solving problems, negotiating or managing conflicts. Although scoring within the mild–WNL range, these patients still had difficulty with daily tasks such as reading train timetables, understanding conversations, interpreting the newspaper or understanding explanations around test results or recommendations provided by their doctor. This subgroup required more extensive testing of higher level language and cognitive communication skills.

Differences between hospital sites were demonstrated within this data sample. JHH is primarily an acute hospital which takes more severely ill patients whereas Belmont Hospital is a district hospital that takes more stable acute patients and sub-acute patients. Patients from BDH had an increased number of speech pathology contacts, increased amounts of therapy and greater length of stay (LOS).

In comparison with Lalor et al.'s (2004) study and Enderby and Petheram (2002), a high proportion of patients received language therapy within this current data sample. This to some extent confirms that speech pathology treatment of aphasia can be achieved within the acute setting concurrently with dysphagia management. It is possible that provision of treatment can be influenced by individual department prioritisation systems as well as patient treatment needs or potential for recovery. Suggestions for patient-based changes in prioritisation and management systems within acute speech pathology are also advocated by Armstrong (2003) and McCooey-O'Halloran et al. (2004). Consideration is also required in regards to growing research suggesting that more intense aphasia therapy, ideally daily, during the acute phase is found to be more effective in improving aphasia post-stroke. This research is demonstrating overall improvements in language recovery when intense and increased hours of therapy are provided during this crucial acute period post-stroke, and is consistent with neuroplasticity principles. Such growing empirical evidence surrounding intensive therapy within this acute period may not only result in significant improvements to the individual's language skills but may improve the individual's ability to participate in rehabilitation programs and potentially reduce anxiety, frustration and depression. Furthermore, targeting aphasia intensely within the acute phase may result in more lifelong improvements in language and everyday communication skills, enhancing quality of life. However, daily therapy was not provided during this timeframe.

Limitations

Some of the limitations of the current project were inherent in the BEST-2 assessment tool. The BEST-2 is not designed to identify high-level language deficits. Further testing was required for this subgroup, as shown by the large amount of patients that fell within the normal to mild range on the BEST-2 but still demonstrated mild aphasia or cognitive communication problems. In addition the BEST-2 does not contain a writing assessment subtest, hence this communicative modality was not included in the assessment data. However, writing should be assessed as part of an aphasia assessment. The authors of the BEST-2 caution that it is a screening tool designed to determine who does have and who does not have aphasia. Further formal diagnostic testing is recommended in order to determine the language area of breakdown and to devise a comprehensive intervention plan.

In some cases there was a delay between admission to hospital and administration of the BEST-2. Factors that limited early administration of the BEST-2 included medical complications, patient drowsiness and being able to access the patient for assessment.

Data collection and analysis involving the Oxfordshire classification and handedness were incomplete. Although there was a statistical difference between Oxfordshire classifications and BEST-2 scores, results could not be analysed for the entire sample. In regards to aphasia therapy provided, the recommended benchmark of daily therapy (Godecke et al. 2008) was not achieved across the two hospitals.

Conclusions

In summary, this data-mining project provided a profile of aphasia language deficits and speech pathology treatment and management in two acute hospital settings. It has demonstrated that speech pathology assessment and treatment of aphasia can be achieved within the acute phase in conjunction with dysphagia management. It also confirms that equal prioritisation of dysphagia and language assessment and treatment post-brain injury is achievable. With growing empirical evidence emerging to support the effectiveness of intense treatment of aphasia in the acute phase, future speech pathology management of this population may require change, perhaps in regards to prioritisation systems and increased staffing ratios. Ongoing research assessing the benefits of early aphasia therapy in the acute model is required to guide appropriate resource allocation in stroke rehabilitation.

Aphasia can have shocking and profoundly negative consequences for individual patients and their families. Patients who were previously high-functioning and independent may suddenly no longer be able to communicate even their most basic needs. Family and staff may erroneously assume the individual has lost their capacity to think for themselves and treat the individual as though they are hearing or cognitively impaired. Although the presence of aphasia may not seem a high priority for healthcare policymakers, the importance of intervention for these patients cannot be underestimated.

Acknowledgements

The authors would like to thank Elisha Cooper, former speech pathologist at John Hunter Hospital, for assistance with data collation. The authors would also like to acknowledge the speech pathologists at John Hunter Hospital for data collected during administration of the BEST-2 tool.

References

Armstrong A (2003). Communication culture in acute speech pathology setting: current issues. *Advances in Speech-Language Pathology,* 5(2): 137–43.

Bakheit AMO, Shaw S, Carrington S & Griffiths S (2007). The rate and extent of improvement with therapy from the different types of aphasia in the first year after stroke. *Clinical Rehabilitation,* 21: 941–49.

Bamford J, Dennis M, Sandercock P, Burn J & Warlow C (1990). The frequency, causes and timing of death within 30 days of a first stroke: the Oxfordshire Community Stroke Project. *Journal of Neurology Neurosurgery and Psychiatry,* 53(10): 824–29.

Bhogal SK, Teasell R, Speechley M & Albert ML (2003). Intensity of aphasia therapy, impact on recovery. *Stroke,* 34: 987–92.

Brady KH & Enderby P (2010). Speech and language therapy for aphasia following stroke. *Cochrane Database Systematic Review,* 12: 5 CD000425.

Burns MS (2008). Application of neuroscience to technology in stroke rehabilitation. *Stroke Rehabilitation,* 15(6): 570–79.

Chapey R (1986). *Language intervention strategies in adult aphasia.* 2nd edn. New York: Williams & Wilkins.

Davies GA (2000). *Aphasiology: disorders & clinical practice.* Boston: Allyn & Bacon.

Enderby P & Petheram B (2002). Has aphasia therapy been swallowed up? *Clinical Rehabilitation,* 16: 604–08.

Engelter ST, Gostynski M, Papa S, Frei M, Born C, Ajdacic-Gross V, Gutzwiller F & Lyrer PA (2006). Epidemiology of aphasia attributable to first ischaemic stroke: incidence, severity, fluency, etiology and thrombolysis. *Stroke,* 37: 1379–84.

Epstein I (2010). *Clinical data-mining: integrating practice and research.* New York: Oxford University Press.

Godecke E, Hird K & Lalor E (2008). Aphasia therapy in the acute setting: is it justified? Paper presented at the Stroke Society of Australasia 2008 Annual Scientific Meeting & Smart Strokes Conference. *Internal Medicine Journal,* 38(Suppl. 4): A71.

Greener J, Enderby P & Whurr R (2000). Speech and language therapy for aphasia following stroke. *Cochrane Database Systematic Review,* 2: CD000425.

Holland A & Fridrikkson J (2001). Aphasia management during the early phases of recovery following stroke. *American Journal of Speech-Language Pathology,* 10(1): 19–28.

Lalor E & Cranfield E (2004). Aphasia: a description of the incidence and management in the acute hospital setting. *Asia Pacific Journal of Speech, Language and Hearing,* 9: 129–36.

Laska AC, Kahan T, Hellblom A, Murray V & von Arbin M (2008). Design and methods of a randomized controlled trial on early speech and language therapy in patients with acute stroke and aphasia. *Topics in Stroke Rehabilitation,* 15(3): 256–61.

McCooey-O'Halloran R, Worrall L & Hickson L (2004). Evaluating the role of speech-language pathology with patients with communication disability in the acute care hospital setting using the ICF. *Journal of Medical Speech-Language Pathology,* 12(2): 49–58.

National Stroke Foundation (NSF) (2009). Facts, figures and statistics. [Online]. Available: www.strokefoundation.com.au/facts-figures-and-stats [Accessed 10 February 2009].

Peach RK (2001). Further thoughts regarding management of acute aphasia following stroke. *American Journal of Speech-Language Pathology,* 10(1): 29–36.

West JF, Sands ES & Ross-Swain D (1988). *The Bedside Evaluation Screening Test for Aphasia (BEST-2).* Austin, Texas: Pro-Ed.

Chapter 8

Unravelling low back pain in an outpatient physiotherapy service

Chris Barnett, Judith Henderson, Robin Haskins, Carla Dyson and Peter Osmotherly

Low back pain (LBP) is a common and costly condition and represents a large proportion of the patient population accessing physiotherapy services. This project used data-mining methodology to investigate the diagnostic and treatment codes used by physiotherapists in the management of low back pain patients and evaluated the reliability and the perceived utility of a relatively new classification system. Further, the clinical outcomes of a cohort of low back pain patients were prospectively evaluated.

Thirteen different low back pain diagnostic codes were used by physiotherapists, with the large majority coded simply as 'low back pain'. Clinician agreement with the new classification system was almost perfect ($\kappa = 0.84$) and largely perceived to be useful. Low back pain patients achieved a clinically important mean change in disability score, with patients classified as 'acute' and 'disc' achieving a greater magnitude of improvement compared to patients classified as 'chronic' and 'non-disc' respectively.

Key words: low back pain, data mining, coding, classification

Low back pain (LBP) is a common presentation to primary and tertiary healthcare centres and was anecdotally a frequent occasion of service within the Royal Newcastle Centre (RNC) and Belmont District Hospital (BDH). Patients with low back pain can utilise high amounts of health resources (Walker et al. 2003), commonly complain of prolonged periods of pain and disability (Waddell 2004) and are often unemployed due to their condition (Maniadakis & Gray 2000).

Low back pain is thought of as not one condition but comprises many discrete classifiable subgroups (Fritz et al. 2007; McKenzie & May 2003; O'Sullivan 2000; Petersen et al. 2003). Emerging evidence suggests that the use of classification systems for non-specific low back pain (NSLBP) to direct treatment is associated with better long-term outcomes (Brennan et al. 2006; Fritz et al. 2003; Kent & Keating 2004; Long et al. 2004).

This project used data-mining methodology to investigate low back pain in patients attending physiotherapy outpatient departments in a public healthcare setting within New South Wales, Australia. Data mining was a design of convenience to fit in with the service needs, which matched the research needs of the department. Despite the limitations of data mining, a practice-based research (PBR) approach (Epstein & Blumenfield 2001) was used to determine important clinical practices concerning classification and treatment of low back pain within our environment.

Many public hospitals within New South Wales, Australia, use the Allied Health Management Information System (AHMIS) as a database to collect and manage administrative and statistical data within allied health departments.

The AHMIS included International Classification of Diseases – 9 (ICD-9) codes from the World Health Organization with over 30 separate codes for low back pain. These have proved cumbersome for physiotherapy practice evaluation in our clinic. The current data-mining project aimed to retrospectively investigate the existing departmental practices and service delivery to this patient population, and trial a novel classification system for low back pain.

Literature review

Low back pain (LBP) is one of the most common and costly conditions managed by health professionals with total estimated health costs of $9.17 billion in Australia in 2001 (Walker et al. 2003). It has a lifetime prevalence of 65 to 80% (Andersson, 1998; Riihimaki 1996) and it is one of the most common conditions presenting to outpatient physiotherapy departments in Australia.

Following the first episode of low back pain, an individual has a 40 to 60% chance of having continued pain and disability after twelve weeks (Abbott & Mercer 2002; Henschke et al. 2008). Consequently, around 15% of the Australian population are reported to suffer from low back pain at any given time (Walker 1999). This high prevalence arguably contributes to low back pain being the most common reason for presenting to general practitioners in Australia (Britt et al. 2009).

Low back pain can have a readily identifiable patho-anatomical cause such as fracture, tumour or inflammatory arthritis but these specific presentations are less common, accounting for fewer than 15% of all low back pain (Deyo & Phillips 1996). Another diagnostic triage category according to clinical practice guidelines is lumbar radiculopathy which is evidence of a neurological conduction deficit. This accounts for approximately 4% of low back pain presentations (Koes et al. 2001) with the remaining majority commonly referred to as non-specific low back pain (NSLBP). The patho-anatomical origin of NSLBP can be difficult to ascertain due to the lack of validity of current diagnostic procedures (Deyo & Phillips 1996; Deyo & Weinstein 2001).

The classification and coding of low back pain and in particular NSLBP has been researched and discussed in the literature at length (Billis et al. 2007; Petersen et al. 1999; Riddle 1998; Spitzer 1987). Indeed Kent and Keating (2004) used qualitative interview methods to ascertain that primary care clinicians believe that NSLBP pain is not one homogenous group but discrete subgroups. However, to date, there is no one universally accepted classification system, despite numerous systems being proposed (Delitto et al. 1995; Fritz et al. 2007; McKenzie & May 2003; O'Sullivan 2005; Petersen et al. 2003).

The Petersen Classification System (PCS) is a relatively new system that aims to identify relevant subgroups of NSLBP utilising the best available evidence for a clinical patho-anatomic orientated diagnostic system (Petersen et al. 2003; Petersen et al. 2004). Aspects of the physiotherapy history and physical examination are used to determine

191

the appropriate classification with no dependence upon imaging or advanced diagnostic procedures. A previous study using four trained physiotherapists investigated the inter-rater reliability of the PCS on a sample of 90 patients with NSLBP. The overall level of agreement was 72% with a substantial chance-corrected degree of agreement ($\kappa = 0.62$) (Petersen et al. 2004).

Identifying subgroups of patients with NSLBP is thought to help match patients to targeted treatments, which may result in improved patient outcomes. Emerging evidence suggests that patient characteristics and assessment findings may help clinicians predict clinically meaningful improvements in disability in response to treatments such as stabilisation exercises (Hicks et al. 2005), spinal manipulation (Flynn et al. 2002, Childs et al. 2004, Hancock et al. 2008) and traction (Cai et al. 2009). Researchers continue to investigate for which patients, under what circumstances, certain treatments may or may not be effective (Kraemer et al. 2002, Stanton et al. 2010).

With regards to NSLBP treatment, clinical practice guidelines recommend providing adequate information and advice, using an active approach and increasing activities gradually to enable patients to take control of their back pain (Bekkering et al. 2003). Patients treated within the clinical practice guidelines tend to achieve better outcomes and incur reduced costs relative to patients treated with modalities not consistent with practice guideline recommendations (Fritz et al. 2007).

Aims of the study

1. To describe our current practice for managing low back pain in a sample of NSW public hospital physiotherapy departments (phase A)

2. To investigate the diagnostic codes used in classifying patients with low back pain (phase A)

3. To analyse treatment codes used in classifying patients with low back pain (phase A)

4. To evaluate the reliability and perceived utility of the Petersen Classification System (PCS) within the department (phase B and C)

5. To measure changes in disability status for a sample of patients with low back pain and to investigate subgroup differences (phase C).

Methodology

Phase A (AHMIS LBP data mining)

A review of existing departmental practices concerning the diagnostic and treatment coding of low back pain patients was conducted using a retrospective analysis of AHMIS data over a two year period.

Phase B (vignette analysis)

Five physiotherapists (experience ranging from one to 15 years) were trained in the use of the PCS via a series of workshops and the dissemination of supporting literature. Case studies (each 2–3 pages in length) were developed by senior clinicians outlining the history and physical examinations findings of five discrete low back pain presentations. Each case study was written to reflect one of the nine mutually exclusive primary sub-classifications within the PCS (see Appendix 1). The five separate case studies were then completed to assess the degree of inter-rater reliability (Siegel & Castellan Jr 1988). Common areas of disagreement were also investigated.

Phase C (Petersen Classification System)

The PCS was trialled in a sample of patients with NSLBP between April and July 2007. Patient demographics were recorded in addition to the measurement of valid and reliable outcomes (See Appendix 1). The primary patient outcome of interest was disability, measured with the Roland-Morris Disability Questionnaire – 18 (RM-18) (Stratford & Binkley 1997). This self-administered tool quantifies the degree of functional restriction, with higher scores reflecting greater levels of disability. A clinically significant change in this scale has been reported as four to five points (Stratford & Binkley 1997; Stratford et al. 1998). The difference between baseline and discharge RM-18 scores was analysed using the t-test for dependent samples.

Differences in the degree of improvement between acute and chronic low back pain and between diagnostic classifications were analysed using tests of interaction in repeated-measures two-way ANOVA with time as the within-subject factor.

Feedback was sought in regards to the perceived clinical utility of this classification system through a survey of participating therapists. Participants were provided with three open-ended questions concerning the feasibility and utility of the PCS and these were returned anonymously (see Appendix 2).

Organisational context

The Royal Newcastle Centre (RNC) is a 144-bed tertiary referral hospital with specialities in: orthopaedics, orthopaedic rehabilitation, rheumatology, urology, ophthalmology, dermatology and immunology. RNC has 6.7 fulltime equivalent staff in outpatient physiotherapy.

The Belmont District Hospital (BDH) is a smaller regional hospital 15 km south of the Royal Newcastle Centre. BDH has 1.2 fulltime equivalent staff in outpatient physiotherapy.

Calvary Mater Newcastle (CMN) is a large tertiary hospital 5 km northeast of the RNC with specialties in oncology and haematology and has an outpatient physiotherapy department with 2.5 fulltime equivalent staff.

Cessnock District Hospital (CDH) is a small regional, rural hospital approximately 30 km from the RNC with an outpatient physiotherapy department staffed by 1.5 fulltime equivalent staff.

Each of these hospitals is located in the eastern sector of Hunter New England Health (HNE), a large metropolitan, regional and rural sector of NSW Health, Australia.

Sample

All patients for both phases A and C were between the ages of 18 and 85 with low back pain as a primary complaint. There were 543 patients in phase A and 41 patients in Phase C.

For Phases B and C, five registered physiotherapists with between one and 15 years clinical experience participated.

Referrals for Phases A and C were received from primary care and community; and hospital specialty teams such as neurosurgery, ortho-paedics and rheumatology.

Data sources and collection process

Phase A (AHMIS LBP data mining)

The AHMIS database was retrospectively mined for all episodes of care at the Royal Newcastle Centre (RNC) and Belmont District Hospital (BDH) departments relating to low back pain between 1 July 2005 and 31 June 2007. All inpatient occasions of service (OOS) were excluded from the dataset, and only patients whose primary code related to low back pain were included.

AHMIS data was converted to a Microsoft Excel spreadsheet to record the patient demographics, treatment codes, wait times and the NSLBP codes physiotherapy that were selected according to the ICD 9. The variables collected included:

1. date of referral received
2. date of initial commencement of episode of care
3. length of treatment episode
4. gender and date of birth
5. medical diagnosis code as per ICD 9
6. treatment codes as per AHMIS.

Phase B (vignette analysis)

Physiotherapists in Royal Newcastle Centre, Belmont District Hospital, Calvary Mater Newcastle (CMN) and Cessnock District Hospital phys-iotherapy departments were trained in the use of the PCS and used six separate case studies (vignette analyses) to assess the degree of clinician reliability.

Completed vignette packages were returned, and clinician agree-ment was determined by calculating the degree of concordance between the multiple raters using the Kappa reliability coefficient for nominal data (Landis & Koch 1977).

Phase C (Petersen Classification System)

A data collection tool was designed to capture the following variables (see Appendix 1):

1. patients subclassification of low back pain as per PCS
2. patient demographics, age, gender
3. duration of LBP
4. change in disability status as measured by the Roland Morris 18 Disability Questionnaire (Stratford & Binkley 1997)
5. treatment utilised.

A one page questionnaire was forwarded to participating therapists, inviting anonymous responses to open-ended questions concerning the clinical utility of the PCS. Feedback was assessed for common themes and trends (see Appendix 2)

Results

Results Phase A: LBP AHMIS data mining

Patient characteristics

During the two year study period a total of 556 patients were treated for low back pain within the RNC and BDH physiotherapy outpatient departments. Of these patients, 302 (54.3%) were female. The mean age of patients was 55.2 years (SD 18.5).

Waiting times

Two hundred and seventy-six patients (49.6%) waited less than one week from the time of referral to their initial consultation. Within two weeks of the referral date 419 patients (75.3%) had commenced episodes of care for NSLBP.

Occasions of service per episode of care

A total of 1,922 occasions of service (OOS) were recorded during the two year period. The mean number of OOS per episode of care for NSLBP patients was 3.5 sessions. Following three OOS, 346 patients

(62.2%) had completed physiotherapy treatment for their back pain. Following six OOS, 498 patients (89.5%) had completed physiotherapy treatment.

Table 8.1: Classification of low back pain as per AHMIS ICD 9 codes

Diagnostic subclassification	Number of patients	Proportion of patients (%)
Low back pain: Discogenic	35	6.3
L/S IVD Disorder	27	4.9
L/S IVD Degeneration	22	4.0
L/S IVD Unspecified Disorder	5	0.9
L/S Canal Stenosis	14	2.5
Low back pain	406	73.0
L/S Sciatica – Neuralgia / Neuritis	5	0.9
L/S Nerve Root Complication / Irritation	11	2.0
L/S Postural Pain, Backache	2	0.4
L/S Instability	10	1.8
L/S Spondylosis Acquired	5	0.9
Sprains & Strains of L/S	7	1.3
L/S: Nerve Root Injury	7	1.3
	556	100

Note. L/S = lumbar spine, IVD = intervertebral disc.

Duration of episodes of care

The duration of each episode of care ranged from 1 to 554 days including one outlier, with an average of 35.3 days (SD 53.5 days). An episode of care was defined as the length between the first recorded occasion of service and the last. Within one week, 157 (28.24%) episodes of care were recorded. By six weeks, episodes of care had been completed for 401 patients (72.2%).

Subclassification of LBP

Thirteen different diagnostic codes were used by physiotherapists for patients presenting with NSLBP (Table 8.1). Across the two year study period 406 patients (73.0%) were coded simply as 'low back pain' and hence not given a specific diagnosis.

Figure 8.1: Treatment codes recorded as per AHMIS for treatment of low back pain

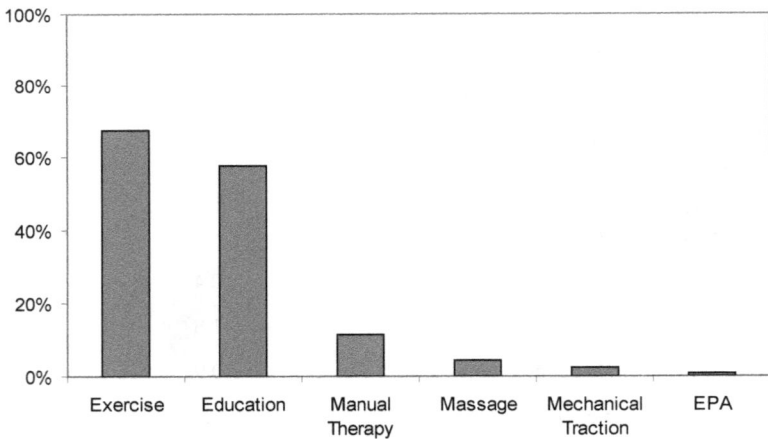

Abbreviations. Manual Therapy = Mobilisation/Manipulation, EPA = Electrotherapy agents such as therapeutic ultrasound.

Treatment interventions

Forty-four separate intervention codes were entered into the AHMIS before being streamlined and organised into seven intervention categories for this study. The most common interventions documented were exercise therapy (67.5%) and patient education (57.6%) (Figure 8.1). Compliance with recording of intervention data by clinicians was high with 93.9% of OOS having interventions entered into the AHMIS system.

Phase B: vignette analysis

Six therapists returned 30 case studies in total. There were no episodes of missing data. Clinician agreement regarding the primary classification for the five vignettes was almost perfect (Landis & Koch 1977), with a Kappa reliability coefficient of 0.84.

On the few episodes of disagreement there was an apparent difficulty in differentiating between the diagnostic classifications 'nerve root entrapment' and 'adherent nerve root'.

Phase C: Petersen Classification System

There were 41 patient records reviewed in this phase of the analysis. Fifty-four percent were female with a mean age of 48.9 years (SD 15.9). The reported median duration of low back pain at the initial consultation was eight weeks (IQR 3-52). The median length of physiotherapy treatment was eight weeks (IQR 6-10). Table 8.2 details the primary diagnostic classifications assigned to patients with low back pain included in this phase of the study.

Patient outcomes: Petersen Classification System

The primary outcome of disability was reported for 93% (n = 38) of baseline participants, however, data was only available for 56% (n = 23) of patients at their final appointment. The mean RM-18 score at baseline was 12.9 (95% CI 10.9-15), and the mean score at discharge was 6.5 (95% CI 4.1-8.8). The mean change score was 6.4 (95% CI 4.2-8.6), which is statistically significant at p <0.001. Seventy percent of the sample achieved a minimal clinically important difference (MCID) in disability at the time of discharge.

Table 8.2: Primary classification of low back pain using the Petersen Classification System

Primary classification	n	%
Disc 1a	13	32%
Disc 1b	2	5%
Disc 1c	8	20%
Adherent nerve root	1	2%
Nerve root entrapment	1	2%
Nerve root compression	0	0%
Stenosis	0	0%
Zygopophyseal joint	8	20%
Postural	0	0%
Sacroiliac joint	1	2%
Dysfunction	3	7%
Inconclusive	4	10%

Acute versus chronic low back pain

Previous research and anecdotal evidence had indicated that patients with acute LBP may experience a greater degree of improvement compared to patients with longer durations of symptoms (Henschke et al. 2008). Data from this sample confirmed this observation with acute patients achieving a larger decrease in RM-18 scores from baseline to discharge compared to patients with chronic LBP ($p = 0.008$).

Seventy-nine percent of acute NSLBP patients in this sample achieved a minimum clinically important difference (MCID) improvement in disability at discharge from physiotherapy treatment. This is in contrast to 56% of the chronic LBP group however this difference was not statistically significant (Fisher's Exact test $p = 0.36$).

Figure 8.2: Pre and post episode of care disability scores for patients with LBP (with 95%CI)

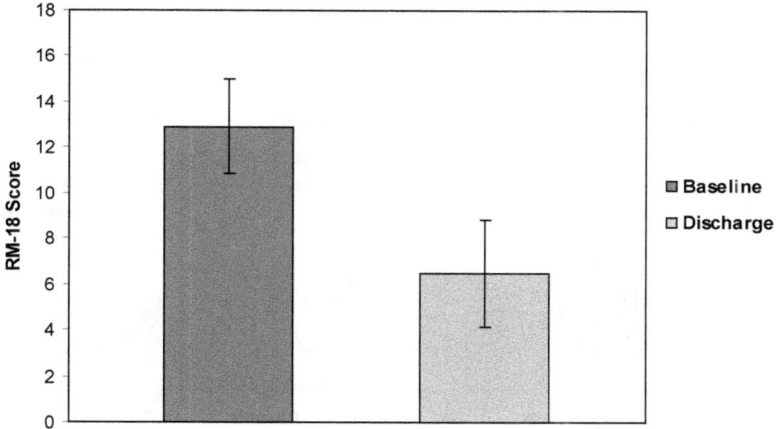

Table 8.3: Comparison of disability scores for acute and chronic low back pain.

	Mean score at baseline (SD)	Mean score at discharge (SD)	Mean score change (95%CI)	P-value (within-group)	P-value (group*time)
Acute LBP (n = 14)	12.29 (5.14)	3.64 (3.8)	8.64 (5.69–11.6)	<0.0001	0.006
Chronic LBP (n = 9)	13.89 (4.96)	10.89 (5.71)	3 (1.08–4.92)	0.007	

Figure 8.3: Histogram comparing disability for acute and chronic LBP

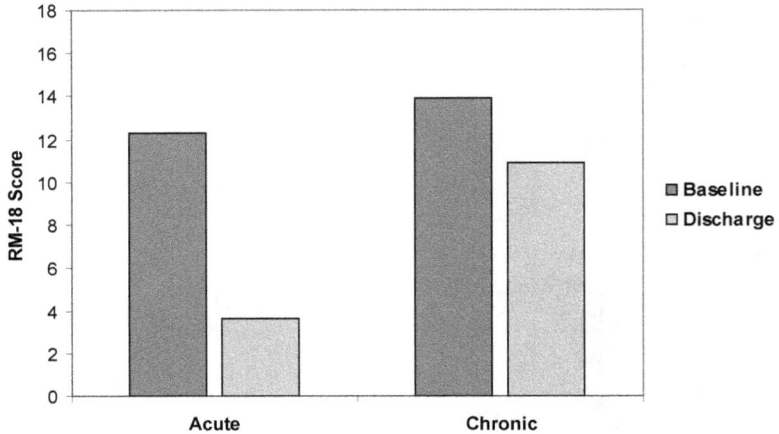

Disc versus non-disc coded patients

Fifty-seven percent of all patients were coded as having disc pathology. Follow up data on disability status was available for approximately half (52%) of this group.

Patients in this dataset classified with the diagnosis of a disc disorder achieved a greater magnitude of improvement in disability from baseline to discharge compared to patients without this classification. This observation trended toward statistical significance ($p = 0.15$).

Ninety-two percent of patients classified as having a disc diagnosis according to the PCS in this sample achieved a MCID improvement in disability at discharge from physiotherapy treatment. This is in contrast to 45% of the patients classified with any other diagnosis. The difference in proportions achieving MCID trended toward statistical significance (Fisher's Exact test $p = 0.063$).

Qualitative feedback for Petersen Classification System (PCS)

Physiotherapists were asked in a brief survey what they thought of the PCS regarding its strengths and weaknesses.

Table 8.4: Comparison of disability between disc and non-disc patients

	Mean score at baseline (SD)	Mean score at discharge (SD)	Mean score change (95% CI)	P-value (within-group)	P-value (group*time)
Disc	15.08 (2.58)	7.17 (5.41)	7.92 (4.9–10.96)	<0.001	0.15
Non-Disc	10.55 (6.02)	5.73 (6.34)	4.82 (1.41–8.23)	0.01	

Figure 8.4: Histogram comparison of disability between disc and non-disc patients

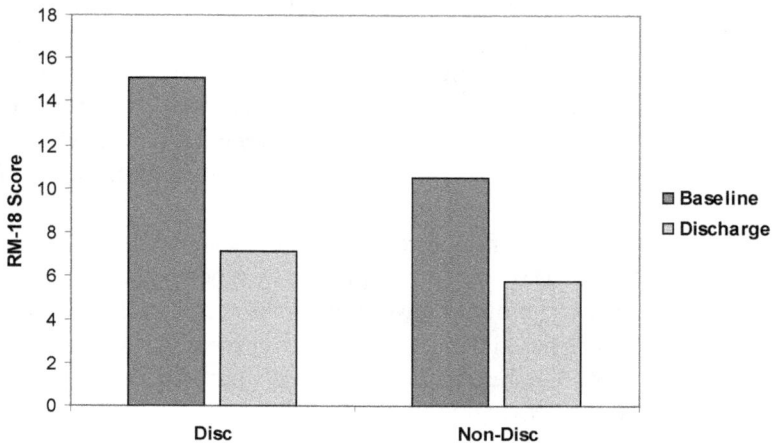

Two key ideas that emerged from the feedback were that clinicians found the tool to be beneficial to their clinical practice and considered it an aid to clinical reasoning.

Clinicians gave feedback that they perceived this classification system was a progression from existing practices, in that it recognised patients with low back pain as a heterogeneous population.

In addition to its use as a diagnostic tool it was believed that it may benefit treatment decision-making.

Discussion

Using data-mining strategies on two separate samples of patients identified with low back pain the department was able to gain a greater depth of understanding about our service for low back pain.

Low back pain was observed to account for over 550 new patients seen within the two year period of audit, which is estimated as approximately 10% of all new referrals to outpatient physiotherapy using our current database. This could be an underestimation of the incidence of low back pain referrals as it excludes patients who had back pain as a secondary complaint which is not recognised by AHMIS.

The AHMIS data reporting that 157 (28.2%) episodes of care were finished at one week is unexpected. The reasons are not known but future data collection on this group may be informative. Access to physiotherapy was prompt with the majority of patients with low back pain seen within two weeks of referral. This is certainly within benchmark for all the department's non urgent patients, who are required to be seen within three weeks for sub-acute and six weeks for chronic conditions.

Our finding of an almost perfect degree of inter-rater reliability (κ = 0.84) using the PCS was higher than previously reported (κ = 0.62) and is most likely the result of our lower number of case samples (5 versus 90) and that paper-based cases were used instead of live patients (Petersen et al. 2004). The results indicate that the participating clinicians were able to sufficiently agree upon the primary classifications in the presented vignettes using the PCS.

The classification of low back pain elicited some interesting results when reviewing the AHMIS data as shown in Table 8.1. The code 'low back pain' was selected 73% in total, perhaps indicating that ICD-9 code-set available for AHMIS entry was deficient for therapist coding needs.

Intervertebral disc disorders contributed to 16.1% of all LBP diagnostic codes, making it the most common specific diagnosis. This finding is consistent with previous research indicating that the intervertebral disc is a common source of NSLBP (Laslett et al. 2006; Laslett et al. 2005; Schwarzer et al. 1995).

When physiotherapists were encouraged to select a specific diagnosis of low back pain using the PCS, once again the discal pathology was the most common patho-anatomical diagnosis, accounting for a much greater 57% of cases followed by facet joint mediated pain at 20%. There were no cases of lumbar stenosis despite the literature reporting a prevalence of 5 to 10% of all low back pain (Watters et al. 2008). This under-representation of stenosis within our sample may be due to the relatively low sample size, or referrer bias with patients with lumbar stenosis commonly being referred for specialist opinion.

When surveying the physiotherapists using the PCS system, it was reported that clinicians perceived that the use of a systematic assessment tool was beneficial to their practice with some citing it as an aid to their diagnostic clinical reasoning. It was noted that many of the surveyed physiotherapists perceived that the PCS may inform their treatment decision making, although it is acknowledged that this is beyond the intended scope of this tool.

Although a large range of treatment codes were available to choose from in the AHMIS database, clinicians appear to have utilised and recorded predominantly exercise and education-based modalities. This trend is also seen from the PCS data. Clinical practice guidelines suggest that *active* treatments such as advice and exercise and empowerment to self-manage should be included in the treatment approach (Fritz et al. 2007; Koes et al. 2001). Electrotherapy and massage were far less prevalent in both datasets, also in agreement with evidence-based practice and clinical guidelines (Koes et al. 2001).

For patients with completed data, the results of our PCS data mining has demonstrated that this group of patients achieves considerable improvements in their perceived disability throughout their episode of care. A mean change of 6.4 on the Roland Morris scale with a lower boundary of the 95% confidence interval of 4.2 suggests that this degree of change is clinically important.

When reviewing acute and chronic low back pain and their disability status, a clear difference in the response was observed, with acute low back pain patients achieving a much larger improvement over time, as compared to those with chronic low back pain. Previous research is consistent with these findings, and this may have implications for physiotherapists providing advice to patients for expected prognosis for low back pain (Henschke et al. 2008).

As seen in the results, patients who were classified as a discal pathology patient by way of the PCS had higher disability scores at baseline but made greater changes in disability compared to non-disc patients over their period of care. Further investigation into whether higher baseline disability scores are associated with disc presentations could be required, and more work is needed in larger populations to confirm this finding. The group of patients with non-disc pathology diagnoses is certainly heterogenous and it is plausible that different classifications of patients within this non-disc sample may have achieved differing magnitudes of improvement. For example, it is not known if those classified with a sacro-iliac joint classification do better or worse than those with a facet joint diagnosis.

Limitations

Datasets are no more reliable that the clinicians entering the data. The AHMIS dataset relies on clinicians' accurately entering data as per department protocols, but it is possible that there is some erroneous data entered. The very short wait times and short treatment times do appear plausible and ongoing audits of wait times are being undertaken and utilized to verify the results. Improved wait list management strategies as described in Chapter 1, and improved GNAHN Physiotherapy staffing levels could have contributed to the very short wait times for physiotherapy outpatients. Physiotherapy staffing levels in Greater Newcastle Area Health network have significantly improved since new measures in recruitment and retention began in 2003.

A lack of reliable and valid outcome measures in AHMIS could be considered a great limitation of the dataset. However, Grimmer et al. (2004) discuss the importance of 'process data' relating to the quality of the patient journey and it is possible that the data-mining methods used recognise more process data than outcome data.

Our study on the PCS showed that the majority of patients with low back pain significantly improved over time; however, cause and effect relations cannot be ascertained from data mining, and a controlled clinical trial would be required if the department was interested in knowing what treatments work best for different types of back pain.

Missing follow up data for the PCS was high at approximately 40%. High attrition rates may bias the final conclusions as the outcome of these patients remains unknown.

The small sample size for the PCS data would limit the internal and external validity of the data. It is also possible that the completed outcome data were open to bias and those patients with a favourable result were more likely to complete treatment and have follow-up data.

The suggestion that patients who are classified as having a discal pathology under the PCS are generally more disabled as compared to non-disc may also be misleading due to the small sample size and the potential for random error. However, this study may provide some preliminary data on the classification of LBP and its natural course.

Conclusions

Using two complementary methods of data mining we have demonstrated a large volume of low back pain patients in our health service are seen within a short waiting time (55% within two weeks), and treated over a short period of time (average treatment time 35 days).

The PCS sample showed that on average patients have significantly reduced disability after physiotherapy treatment, especially for acute low back pain. The mean change score for disability for all low back pain was 6.4 on the RM-18 which is a clinically meaningful difference (Stratford & Binkley 1997).

Our data did not suggest any difference in pain and disability between classification codes for the Petersen sample, but patients who were grouped together as discogenic appear to have higher initial levels of disability and a trend towards a greater improvement in disability over time as compared to non-disc patients.

The dilemma concerning accurate and reliable coding of low back pain continues, with discussion and diverse views being expressed in current literature. There has been a recent move away from patho-anatomical models towards treatment-based classifications (Fritz 2009; Hancock et al. 2009) and those concerning movement impairment and biopsychosocial models (O'Sullivan 2005).

A new coding set could be recommended on the basis of the current clinical guidelines which currently recommend triaging all low back pain into specific pathologies such as fracture or tumour, for example, followed by radiculopathy, and subsequently NSLBP.

Data mining has proved a suitable methodology for practice-based research, that has allowed us to reflect upon a large volume of data and draw meaningful conclusions that will inform departmental practices and guide potential research agenda.

Acknowledgements

Belmont District Hospital, Calvary Mater Newcastle and Cessnock District Hospital Physiotherapy Departments.

References

Abbott J & Mercer S (2002). The natural history of acute low back pain. *New Zealand Journal of Physiotherapy,* 30(3): 8–16.

Andersson GB (1998). Epidemiology of low back pain. *Acta Orthopaedica Scandinavica Supplementum,* 281: 28–31.

Bekkering GE, Hendriks HJM, Koes BW, Oostendorp RAB, Ostelo RWJG, Thomassen JMC & van Tulder MW (2003). Dutch physiotherapy guidelines for low back pain. *Physiotherapy,* 89(2): 82–96.

Billis EV, McCarthy CJ & Oldham JA (2007). Subclassification of low back pain: a cross-country comparison. *European Spine Journal,* 16(7): 865–79.

Brennan GP, Fritz JM, Hunter SJ, Thackeray A, Delitto A & Erhard RE (2006). Identifying subgroups of patients with acute/subacute 'nonspecific' low back pain: results of a randomized clinical trial. *Spine,* 31(6): 623–31.

Britt H, Miller GC, Charles J, Henderson J, Bayram C, Pan Y, Valenti L, Harrison C, Fahridin S & O'Halloran J (2009). General practice activity in Australia 2008–09. [Online]. Available: www.aihw.gov.au/publication-detail/?id=6442468308 [Accessed 28 April 2011].

Cai C, Pua YH & Lim KC (2009). A clinical prediction rule for classifying patients with low back pain who demonstrate short-term improvement with mechanical lumbar traction. *European Spine Journal*, 18(4): 554–61.

Childs JD, Fritz JM, Flynn TW, Irrgang JJ, Johnson KK, Majkowski GR & Delitto A (2004). A clinical prediction rule to identify patients with low back pain most likely to benefit from spinal manipulation: a validation study. *Annals of Internal Medicine*, 141(12): 920–28.

Delitto A, Erhard RE & Bowling RW (1995). A treatment-based classification approach to low back syndrome: identifying and staging patients for conservative treatment. *Physical Therapy*, 75(6): 470–85.

Deyo RA & Phillips WR (1996). Low back pain: a primary care challenge. *Spine*, 21(24): 2826–32.

Deyo RA & Weinstein JN (2001). Low back pain. *New England Journal of Medicine*, 344(5): 363–70.

Epstein I & Blumenfield S (2001). *Clinical data-mining in practice-based research: social work in hospital settings.* New York: Haworth Social Work Practice Press.

Flynn T, Fritz J, Whitman J, Wainner R, Magel J, Rendeiro D, Butler B, Garber M & Allison S (2002). A clinical prediction rule for classifying patients with low back pain who demonstrate short-term improvement with spinal manipulation. *Spine*, 27(24): 2835–43.

Fritz JM (2009). Clinical prediction rules in physical therapy: coming of age? *Journal of Orthopaedic and Sports Physical Therapy*, 39(3): 159–61.

Fritz JM, Cleland JA & Brennan GP (2007). Does adherence to the guideline recommendation for active treatments improve the quality of care for patients with acute low back pain delivered by physical therapists? *Medical Care*, 45(10): 973–80.

Fritz JM, Cleland JA & Childs JD (2007). Subgrouping patients with low back pain: evolution of a classification approach to physical therapy. *Journal of Orthopaedic and Sports Physical Therapy,* 37(6): 290–302.

Fritz JM, Delitto A & Erhard RE (2003). Comparison of classification-based physical therapy with therapy based on clinical practice guidelines for patients with acute low back pain: a randomized clinical trial. *Spine,* 28(13): 1363–71.

Grimmer K, Bialocerkowski A, Kumar S & Milanese S (2004). Implementing evidence in clinical practice: the 'therapies' dilemma. *Physiotherapy,* 90(4): 189–94.

Hancock M, Herbert RD & Maher CG (2009). A guide to interpretation of studies investigating subgroups of responders to physical therapy interventions. *Physical Therapy,* 89(7): 698–704.

Hancock MJ, Maher CG, Latimer J, Herbert RD & McAuley JH (2008). Independent evaluation of a clinical prediction rule for spinal manipulative therapy: a randomised controlled trial. *European Spine Journal,* 17(7): 936–43.

Henschke N, Maher CG, Refshauge KM, Herbert RD, Cumming RG, Bleasel J, York J, Das A & McAuley J (2008). Prognosis in patients with recent onset low back pain in Australian primary care: inception cohort study. *British Medical Journal,* 337(7662): 154–57.

Hicks GE, Fritz JM, Delitto A & McGill SM (2005). Preliminary development of a clinical prediction rule for determining which patients with low back pain will respond to a stabilization exercise program. *Archives of Physical Medicine and Rehabilitation,* 86(9): 1753–62.

Kent P & Keating J (2004). Do primary-care clinicians think that nonspecific low back pain is one condition? *Spine,* 29(9): 1022–31.

Koes BW, van Tulder MW, Ostelo R, Burton AK & Waddell G (2001). Clinical guidelines for the management of low back pain in primary care: an international comparison. *Spine,* 26(22): 2504–13.

Kraemer HC, Wilson GT, Fairburn CG & Agras WS (2002). Mediators and moderators of treatment effects in randomized clinical trials. *Archives of General Psychiatry,* 59(10): 877–83.

Landis JR & Koch GG (1977). The measurement of observer agreement for categorical data. *Biometrics,* 33(1): 159–74.

Laslett M, Aprill CN, McDonald B & Oberg B (2006). Clinical predictors of lumbar provocation discography: a study of clinical predictors of lumbar provocation discography. *European Spine Journal,* 15(10): 1473–84.

Laslett M, Oberg B, Aprill CN & McDonald B (2005). Centralization as a predictor of provocation discography results in chronic low back pain, and the influence of disability and distress on diagnostic power. *Spine Journal: Official Journal of the North American Spine Society,* 5(4): 370–80.

Long A, Donelson R & Fung T (2004). Does it matter which exercise? A randomized control trial of exercise for low back pain. *Spine,* 29(23): 2593–602.

Maniadakis N & Gray A (2000). The economic burden of back pain in the UK. *Pain,* 84(1): 95–103.

McKenzie R & May S (2003). *The lumbar spine: mechanical diagnosis and therapy.* Waikanae: Spinal Publications New Zealand Ltd.

O'Sullivan P (2005). Diagnosis and classification of chronic low back pain disorders: maladaptive movement and motor control impairments as underlying mechanism. *Manual Therapy,* 10(4): 242–55.

Petersen T, Laslett M, Thorsen H, Manniche C, Ekdahl C & Jacobsen S (2003). Diagnostic classification of non-specific low back pain. A new system integrating patho-anatomic and clinical categories. *Physiotherapy Theory and Practice,* 19(4): 213–37.

Petersen T, Olsen S, Laslett M, Thorsen H, Manniche C, Ekdahl C & Jacobsen S (2004). Inter-tester reliability of a new diagnostic classification system for patients with non-specific low back pain. *Australian Journal of Physiotherapy,* 50(2): 85–91.

Petersen T, Thorsen H, Manniche C & Ekdahl C (1999). Classification of nonspecific low back pain: a review of the literature on classification systems relevant to physiotherapy. *Physical Therapy Reviews,* 4: 265–81.

Riddle DL (1998). Classification and low back pain: a review of the literature and critical analysis of selected systems. *Physical Therapy,* 78(7): 708–37.

Riihimaki H (1996). Epidemiology and pathogenesis of non-specific low back pain: what does the epidemiology tell us? *Bulletin of the Hospital for Joint Diseases,* 55(4): 197–98.

Schwarzer AC, Aprill CN, Derby R, Fortin J, Kine G & Bogduk N (1995). The prevalence and clinical features of internal disc disruption in patients with chronic low back pain. [Research Support, Non-U.S. Gov't]. *Spine,* 20(17): 1878–83.

Siegel S & Castellan Jr NJ (1988). *Nonparametric statistics for the behavioral sciences.* New York: McGraw-Hill Book Company.

Spitzer WO (1987). Chapter 3: diagnosis of the problem (The problem of diagnosis). *Spine,* 12(S16–S21).

Stanton TR, Hancock MJ, Maher CG & Koes BW (2010). Critical appraisal of clinical prediction rules that aim to optimize treatment selection for musculoskeletal conditions. *Physical Therapy,* 90(6): 843–54.

Stratford PW & Binkley JM (1997). Measurement properties of the RM-18: a modified version of the Roland-Morris disability scale. *Spine,* 22(20): 2416–21.

Stratford PW, Binkley JM, Riddle DL & Guyatt GH (1998). Sensitivity to change of the Roland-Morris Back Pain Questionnaire: part 1. [Research Support, Non-U.S. Gov't]. *Physical Therapy,* 78(11): 1186–96.

Waddell G (2004). *The back pain revolution.* 2nd edn. Edinburgh: Churchill Livingstone.

Walker BF (1999). The prevalence of low back pain in Australian adults. A systematic review of the literature from 1966–1998. *Asia-Pacific Journal of Public Health,* 11(1): 45–51.

Walker BF, Muller R & Grant WD (2003). Low back pain in Australian adults: the economic burden. *Asia-Pacific Journal of Public Health,* 15(2): 79–87.

Watters WC 3rd, Baisden J, Gilbert TJ, Kreiner S, Resnick DK, Bono CM, Ghiselli G, Heggeness MH, Mazanec DJ, O'Neill C, Reitman CA, Shaffer WO, Summers JT, Toton JF & North American Spine Society (2008). Degenerative lumbar spinal stenosis: an evidence-based clinical guideline for the diagnosis and treatment of degenerative lumbar spinal stenosis. *Spine Journal: Official Journal of the North American Spine Society,* 8(2): 305–10.

Appendix 1: Petersen Classification System data collection sheet

PHYSIOTHERAPY DEPARTMENT
LBP DATA COLLECTION SHEET

HUNTER NEW ENGLAND
NSW⊕HEALTH

Therapist: _____

Site: _____

Patient Sticker

Commencement of episode of care: _____(date)

Approximate duration of symptoms this episode: _____(years, months, weeks)

Related symptoms this episode: ☐ Pain between T_{12} and gluteal folds
(tick all that apply)   ☐ Pain between gluteal folds and knees
                                                    ☐ Pain below knees
                                                    ☐ Paraesthesia

Petersen Classification
Using the Petersen classification system, please indicate the relevant diagnostic categories (note that categories 1-9 are mutually exclusive, however they may coexist with categories 10 to 12).

- ☐ 1. Disc Syndrome (please indicate one of the following 3 subcategories)
    - o   mechanical reducible disc
    - o   mechanical irreducible disc
    - o   non-mechanical disc
- ☐ 2. Adherent Nerve Root Syndrome
- ☐ 3. Nerve Root Entrapment Syndrome
- ☐ 4. Nerve Root Compression Syndrome
- ☐ 5. Spinal Stenosis Syndrome
- ☐ 6. Zygapophysial Joint Syndrome
- ☐ 7. Postural Syndrome
- ☐ 8. Sacroiliac Joint Syndrome
- ☐ 9. Dysfunction Syndrome
- ☐ 10. Myofascial Pain Syndrome
- ☐ 11. Adverse Neural Tension Syndrome
- ☐ 12. Abnormal Pain Syndrome
- ☐ 13. Inconclusive

OUTCOME MEASURE	BASELINE: DATE	DISCHARGE: DATE
RM-18		*Insert NA if not possible to obtain (eg. DNA)*
Other		*Insert NA if not possible to obtain (eg. DNA)*
Other		*Insert NA if not possible to obtain (eg. DNA)*

Treatment Plan (eg. McKenzie, graded exposure etc.): _____

_____

Additional Comments: _____

Appendix 2: Survey to evaluate Petersen Classification System

COMMENTS

Please provide any comments you have regarding the use a data code set that identifies classifications of low back pain for data mining purposes.

_____
_____
_____
_____
_____
_____

Please provide any comments you have regarding the Petersen Classification System as a method for sub-classification of non-specific low back pain.

_____
_____
_____
_____
_____
_____
_____

Please provide any additional comments

_____
_____
_____
_____

Thank you for taking the time to complete the case studies and providing your comments. Please return the completed package to Robin Haskins or Chris Barnett, Physiotherapy Department, Royal Newcastle Centre.

Chapter 9

Pre-operative assessment of voice abnormalities in patients with thyroid disease: a clinical data-mining exploration of 'thyroid voice'

Sarah L Bone, Anne E Vertigan and Robert L Eisenberg

This chapter describes how clinical data mining (CDM) was used as a research method for investigating the vocal features of patients who have thyroid disease. More specifically, it was used to empirically validate the presence of distinctive vocal features in patients with thyroid disease. Subjects were adult patients who had attended pre-operative voice assessment in the Speech Pathology Department at John Hunter Hospital (JHH) as part of the Hunter Elective Admission Planned Pre-operative Service. Available patient data collected between 2003 and 2007 were extracted and organised by practitioners so that statistical data analysis could be performed. Both the process and findings of this CDM study are presented as well as the potential for future exploration of the data. It was found overall that 80% of patients with thyroid disease presented pre-operatively with voice difficulties or related upper airway symptoms that are associated with voice problems in patients with thyroid disease.

Key words: thyroid disease, voice, dysphonia, otolaryngology, clinical data mining

This clinical data-mining project developed when an otolaryngologist approached a speech pathologist with the idea that there was distinctive entity known as 'thyroid voice'. The otolaryngologist requested speech pathology assessments on patients with thyroid disease. Although many speech pathology texts cite thyroid disease as having an impact on voice (Verdolini et al. 2006; Colton et al. 2006), the concept of a distinct 'thyroid voice' to denote the clinical perception of specific voice changes generally associated with thyroid disease is not universally accepted within the speech pathology community.

A thyroid voice clinic was established in 2003 as a joint venture between the otolaryngologist and speech pathologists. Together they decided to create and store a database of assessment results for each patient seen in the clinic. This database grew into a source of valuable clinical data collected from pre- and post-operative voice assessments suitable for analysis. The thyroid caseload currently makes up a significant portion of the outpatients referred to the Speech Pathology Department at John Hunter Hospital.

In particular, team members wanted to determine whether there were identifiable voice features that were abnormal in patients with various thyroid diseases and what these features were. The otolaryngologists specifically asked the speech pathologists to empirically explore the concept of 'thyroid voice'. Rather than relying on practice wisdom alone, this study sought to determine which types of thyroid disease were associated with voice abnormalities prior to surgical intervention.

With a CDM study possible, these practitioner researchers decided to improve their understanding of pre-operative voice features in patients with thyroid disease with an ultimate desire to improve clinical care for this caseload. They began by conceptualising a study that would answer a number of questions about pre-operative patients.

The role of the thyroid gland in the human body is to regulate protein synthesis and tissue metabolism by producing thyroid hormones. The thyroid hormones are responsible for a number of normal human body functions including maintenance of body temperature and growth, especially the growth of the nervous and skeletal systems (Tortora & Derrickson 2007). Thyroid disease can affect an individual's general health, and can also lead to specific problems of voice production (Sataloff et al. 1997).

Speech pathology is a health profession responsible for the diagnosis, management and treatment of individuals who are unable to communicate effectively or who have difficulty with feeding and swallowing (Speech Pathology Australia Limited 2010). These communication problems can include difficulties with speech, language or voice. Speech pathologists often work with patients with thyroid disease because the voice can be affected as a result of the disease itself or as a consequence of thyroid surgery. It has been suggested in previous literature that speech pathologists should routinely assess the voices of patients who are undergoing thyroid surgery (Hong & Kim 1997) to ensure early diagnosis of voice problems and to ensure early commencement of voice therapy. Pre-operative voice assessment is essential for establishment of baseline, differential diagnosis and measurement of change following surgery.

Hyperthyroidism and hypothyroidism are known aetiologies of organic voice disorders (Aronson & Bless 2009). There are a number of reasons why the voice may change as a result of thyroid disease. These reasons include muscular weakness, submucosal vocal fold changes, unusual sensations in the throat and compression effects of the thyroid gland itself on structures that are used to produce voice. In some cases of hyperthyroidism where thyrotoxicosis occurs, muscular weakness and submucosal changes of the vocal folds may result (Sataloff et al. 1997). Voice disturbances are uncommon in mild hyperthyroidism. In hypothyroidism the fluid content of the vocal fold can be affected leading to increased tissue bulk and mass of the vocal folds (Verdolini et al. 2006; Koschkee & Rammage 1997). This increased bulk and mass of the vocal folds may lead to vocal fatigue, hoarseness of the voice, reduced pitch range and sensations of a lump in the throat. It is believed that in cases of prolonged hypothyroidism, myexedema can result, which causes oedema within subcutaneous tissue in the larynx or elsewhere (Verdolini et al. 2006). However, there are no documented findings regarding the effects of hypothyroidism on the voice (Verdolini et al. 2006).

In addition to the hormonal effects that lead to vocal changes in people with thyroid disease there is also a risk of true vocal fold motion being impaired pre-operatively (Farrag et al. 2006). Voice changes can also occur as a result of structural thyroid disorders such as thyroid goitres, nodules or cancers where there is interference on the larynx or trachea known as compression. Compression refers to the pressure on other vital structures of the neck such as the trachea or oesophagus. Structural changes of the diseased thyroid gland by way of tumour, goitre, thyroiditis or thyrotoxicity can also interfere with voice production by causing vocal fold paralysis or by impairing vertical laryngeal movement (Sataloff et al. 1997). Similarly, surgery to the neck such as thyroidectomy may lead to permanent damage to the vocal mechanism through scarring of the extrinsic laryngeal musculature (Sataloff et al. 1997).

Whilst there is no structural reason to suspect voice alteration in patients with parathyroid disease, the inclusion of this group of patients was requested by the otolaryngologist. The parathyroid glands are located behind or around the thyroid gland and in some rare cases may be located within the thyroid gland itself. The parathyroid glands are involved in the regulation of calcium, phosphate and magnesium in the blood by producing and secreting parathyroid hormone (Tortora & Derrickson 2007). Patients who were scheduled for parathyroid surgery were included in this research project as a comparison group.

Motion of the true vocal folds may be impaired in thyroid disease because of the close anatomic position of the recurrent laryngeal nerve to the thyroid gland. Invasive cancers originating from the thyroid gland or enlargement of the thyroid such as in multinodular goitres (MNG) extending outside into neighbouring anatomy may interfere with the function of the recurrent laryngeal nerve leading to impaired true vocal fold motion (Farrag et al. 2006). Mechanical pressure or straining of the recurrent laryngeal nerve can lead to incomplete paralysis where only some of the motor units are affected. In an incomplete recurrent laryngeal nerve paralysis such as this, the vocal fold may still have mobility but reduced muscular tone, reduced mucosal wave and asymmetrical bilateral waves (Koçak et al. 1999).

It could be proposed that thyroid patients with compressive symptoms may experience anxiety or develop maladaptive vocal behaviours in response to having a mass in the throat (Meek et al. 2008). Medically, there is an association between thyroid function and psychiatric disturbances (Whybrow & Bauer 2000). Psychiatric features associated with thyrotoxicosis include acute or chronic mania, delusions and hallucinations, insanity, melancholia with a tendency for suspicion and self-accusation, agoraphobia, dementia or even suicidal ideation (Whybrow & Bauer 2000). Additionally, Verdolini et al. (2006) describe irritability in patients with hyperthyroidism. There is no literature to support psychogenic factors being associated with voice disorders in patients with thyroid disease. It is intuitively possible that psychosocial factors could affect voice in people with organic voice disorders such as thyroid disease; however, Baker (2008) states that there is a paucity of published data examining psychosocial factors as contributing factors to organic voice disorders.

The majority of previous research in the field of voice and thyroid disease has focused on the prevalence of voice disorders in thyroid patients after their surgery with an emphasis on nerve damage or structural alterations to anatomy related to surgery (Soylu et al. 2007; Debruyne et al. 1997; Hong & Kim 1997; Stojadinovic et al. 2002; Ortega et al. 2008). Despite this, there is limited data on pre-operative vocal features in patients with thyroid disease. Farrag et al. (2006) assessed preoperative vocal fold mobility using indirect mirror laryngoscopy, fibre-optic examination and videostroboscopy. However, it was beyond the scope of this study to include acoustic or auditory perceptual voice measures.

A major limitation of current literature is the lack of detailed exploration of the symptoms and vocal features of patients with specific thyroid diseases and varying compressive status. For the purpose of this CDM study, the focus was to examine specific symptoms and vocal features of patients with different types of thyroid disease prior to their surgery and to determine whether the vocal features are different for patients with compressive versus non-compressive thyroid disease.

Study aims

The aims of the study were to determine the pre-operative vocal features of patients with thyroid and parathyroid disease:

1. identify particular vocal features in patients with specific types of thyroid disease such as multinodular goitres or thyroid cancers
2. examine particular vocal features in patients with compression of the thyroid gland compared to patients who do not have compression of the thyroid gland.

Methodology

This study was conducted within John Hunter Hospital's Speech Pathology Department in association with the otolaryngology surgery team. All referrals were made by an otolaryngologist who is a medical specialist in diseases of the ear, nose and larynx. All participants underwent pre-operative flexible fibre-optic nasendoscopy which was conducted by the otolaryngology surgery team. Referrals detailed the participant's demographic details, thyroid disease diagnosis and compression type.

Thyroid disease diagnosis was classified differentially by the otolaryngologist as (a) parathyroid, (b) multinodular goitre, (c) thyroid cancer, (d) thyroid nodule, (e) toxicity.

Compressive status was classified as: (a) definite compression, (b) possible/early compression, and (c) no compression. This project received a formal waiver from the Hunter Area Research Ethics Committee as not needing to submit the protocol for full ethical review.

Sample

The sample consisted entirely of referred patients who were waiting to undergo thyroid surgery. The range of ages was from 18 to 79 years of age. Participants had a range of thyroid-related diagnoses and compression status. Included in the study were 115 referrals. Out of the 115 referrals, 112 (97%) received a pre-operative voice assessment. Therefore, the original sample size was reduced by three. These patients failed to attend a pre-operative appointment, cancelled their appointment or were unable to obtain an appointment in the clinic prior to their surgery date due to staff leave without backfill.

Data sources and collection process

One hundred and twelve patients included in the study received comprehensive voice assessments. Voice assessments comprised routine clinical care from the Speech Pathology Department. Data collected during each assessment included: (a) self-reported voice and upper airway symptom rating scores calculated from responses to the symptom rating questionnaire (Vertigan et al. 2007), (b) auditory perceptual voice analysis of a connected speech sample, *Grandfather passage* (Darley et al. 1975), (c) acoustic voice assessment using a sustained phonation task on /a/, pitch range task using a stepped pitch range and (d) electroglottographic analysis during passage reading of the *Rainbow passage* (Fairbanks 1960). The specific measures analysed in this project are listed in Table 9.1.

Voice samples were recorded by a Studio Condenser Microphone NT3 (RODE) positioned 10 cm from the mouth and recorded directly into a personal computer. These were recorded in a sound-treated room. The voice recordings were stored on the hard drive of a personal computer in the speech pathology treatment room with a sampling rate of 44.1 kHz. These voice samples were analysed using the PRAAT acoustics program (Boersma 2005) and auditory perceptual voice analysis.

The speech pathologists used the auditory perceptual rating tool Perceptual Voice Profile (Oates & Russell 1998) to analyse the auditory perceptual features of the voices during reading of the *Grandfather passage* (Darley et al. 1975). The Perceptual Voice Profile involves rating sixteen parameters of voice on a scale using the severity of *normal, slight, mild, moderate, moderate–severe* and *severe* for each parameter. These ratings were then converted to a numeric value from *0 = normal* to *6 = severe*. The most severe perceptual features for pitch and quality were used in the final analysis. Formal analysis of the auditory perceptual data was beyond the scope of this project and will be analysed in a separate study. Voice samples were rated by two trained speech pathologists that were blind to the diagnoses and compression status of each patient and were not involved in the patient's assessment appointments. The ratings between the two judges were compared. The judges were in agreement or within plus/minus one point on the six-point rating scale for 1534 (98%) parameters. There was a significant and moderate correlation between the ratings of the two judges (r_s = .604, p < .001). The 18 parameters on which the judges differed were re-rated in a subsequent session where the two speech pathologists conferred to produce a single consensus rating for each of the parameters. The consensus ratings were used in the statistical analysis of the results. Intra-rater reliability was calculated using 20 repeated samples, which were rated twice by each of the two speech pathologists. Intra-rater reliability was 100% for rater one (r_s = .686, p < .001) and 99% for rater two (r_s = .668, p < .001) using the +/– 1 severity scale criterion.

Acoustic analysis was conducted on sustained vowels. These vowels were elicited by instructing participants to take a deep breath in and say /a/ for as long as they possibly could at a comfortable pitch and loudness level (Hirano 1981; Baken & Orlikoff 2000). This task was performed three times.

Electroglottography using the Laryngograph Speech Studio Pty Ltd. was also used to analyse samples of connected speech obtained by reading the extended version of the *Rainbow passage* (Fairbanks 1960).

The results for each patient including age, gender, thyroid disease diagnoses and compressive status, self-reported symptom rating questionnaires, and acoustic, auditory-perceptual and electroglottograph assessments were entered onto three separate Excel database spreadsheets. This data was then transferred to Statistical Package for the Social Sciences (SPSS version 19) for analysis using both one- and two-way ANOVAs and independent *t* tests. The significance level to determine differences between groups was set at p < .05.

Table 9.1: Summary of voice features measured during pre-operative assessment

Assessment	Measure
Symptom frequency and severity rating	Total symptom score
	Breathing score
	Cough score
	Voice score
	Upper airway score
Auditory perceptual features	Overall quality
	Overall pitch
Acoustic measures	Maximum phonation time (seconds)
	Fundamental frequency of sustained vowel (Hertz)
	Standard deviation of fundamental frequency for sustained vowel (Hertz)
	Jitter (%)
	Harmonics-to-noise ratio (dB SPL)
	Phonation frequency range (semitones)
	Fundamental frequency connected speech (Hertz)
Electroglottography	Irregularity of fundamental frequency (%) = CFx
	Irregularity of closed phase cycle of vibration (%) = CQx
	Closed phase cycle of vibration (%) = Qx

Results

Information was collected from 112 participants with a mean age of 51 years (SD = 16) who presented to the thyroid voice assessment clinic. There were 84 female participants (75%) and 28 male participants

(25%). Table 9.2 presents participants classified according to specific thyroid diagnosis. There were 48 participants with multinodular goitre, 27 with a singular thyroid nodule, 16 with thyroid cancer, 15 with parathyroid disease and six with thyroid toxicity (Table 9.2). The participants were also classified by compressive status, defined as compression of the thyroid gland into surrounding anatomical structures in the neck. Forty-five participants had definite compression, 62 had no compression and five had possible or early compression.

Table 9.2: Participant demographics

Diagnostic subgroup	Number	% female	Age (years) M (SD)	% compressive symptoms *
Multinodular goitre	48	40	54 (14)	67 (69)
Thyrotoxic	6	100	46 (19)	0 (0)
Parathyroid	15	53	59 (15)	0 (0)
Cancer	16	56	46 (20)	25 (38)
Nodule	27	70	46 (15)	33 (37)

Note. * = includes patients with both definite, early and possible compressive symptoms; M = mean; SD = standard deviation

Table 9.3 displays pre-operative symptom rating scores according to the participants' diagnostic subgroups. Fifty-eight percent of participants with multinodular goitre had symptom frequency and severity scores outside the normal range. Forty-one percent of participants with nodule and 33% of participants with toxicity had abnormal total symptom scores. Both the cancer and parathyroid groups had 13% of participants with abnormal symptom scores. Upper airway symptoms were most commonly reported by all groups. Participants with multinodular goitre also commonly reported breathing difficulties. The data was normally distributed. Comparison of diagnostic groups using one-way ANOVAs revealed that there was a significant difference between diagnostic groups for breathing (p = 0.009), cough (p = 0.001), upper airway (p = 0.028) and total symptom scores (p = 0.032) but not for voice. Post hoc analysis using the Post Hoc Tukey test revealed that breathing scores were significantly higher in the multinodular group than in the parathyroid group (p = 0.015) although with Bonferroni adjustment (p < .01) this result was not significantly different. Cough scores were significantly higher in the multinodular group than the nodule group (p = 0.007).

Table 9.3: Pre-operative symptom rating scores group by diagnosis

	MNG (n = 48) M (SD)	Cancer (n = 16)M (SD)	Toxicity (n = 6) M (SD)	Nodule (n = 27) M (SD)	Para-thyroid (n = 15) M (SD)	F Value	P value
Total score	20 (15)	15.3 (16)	12.8 (6)	13.8 (17)	6 .3(7)	2.741	0.032*
Breathing	3.9 (4)	1.6 (3)	2.8 (3)	2.1 (3)	0.9 (1.4)	3.540	0.009*
Cough	5.3 (4)	3.9 (3)	4.2 (2)	1.8 (3)	2.7 (2)	4.837	0.001*
Voice	4 (4)	3.9 (6)	1.8 (2)	3.5 (5)	1.5 (2)	1.020	0.401
Upper airway	8.1 (7)	6.7 (7)	5 (4)	5.2 (6)	2.4 (3)	2.836	0.028*

Note. MNG = multinodular goitre; M = mean; SD = standard deviation, * = significant difference

A substantial proportion of patients in each subgroup had abnormal acoustic values; however, these were not universally abnormal (Table 9.4). Maximum phonation time (MPT) is described as the maximum length of time a vowel can be sustained on one breath. A higher value for MPT indicates better performance and values above 15 seconds are considered to be within normal limits (Hirano et al. 1968). Mean fundamental frequency (MFF) is the average number of vibratory cycles per second in the speech sample and for the purpose of this study was measured during sustained phonation. For this study MFF was considered normal if it fell between 101 and 140 Hz for males and between 169 and 241 Hz for females (Baken & Orlikoff 2000). MFF correlates perceptually to pitch. Standard deviation of fundamental frequency of sustained vowels (SD F°) is the variability in fundamental frequency in a single voice sample (Stassen et al. 2005). In this study SD F° was considered normal if it was less than 10 Hz. Jitter of sustained vowels is defined as the mean difference between periods of adjacent cycles divided by the mean period and is therefore a fundamental frequency-related measure (Dejonckere et al. 2001). Jitter indicates the variability of the pitch period within the analysed voice sample and gives an index of stability of the phonatory system (Baken & Orlikoff 2000). Jitter values over 1% are considered pathological according to the PRAAT acoustics program (Boersma 2005). Harmonics-to-noise ratio is a measure of the amount of noise present in the signal (Speyer et al. 2004). It is a ratio of the total energy in the voice signal to the energy in the aperiodic components of voice (Gorham-Rowan 2004). The normative value for harmonics-to-noise ratio (HNR) in this study was 20 dB as per the PRAAT acoustics program (Boersma 2005). Jitter and harmonic-to-noise ratio correlate perceptually to voice quality. Phonation frequency range (PFR) is the difference between the maximum and minimum pitch that can be produced by a speaker. The higher the PFR indicates better performance; however, there is a trend towards reduction of PFR with increased age (Baken & Orlikoff 2000). PFR is said to reflect the physiological limits of the patient's voice and determines certain aspects of the limits of laryngeal adjustments (Colton et al. 2006). For the purpose of this study, PFR was considered normal if it was greater than 13.8 semitones (Vertigan et al. 2008).

Statistical analysis using a one-way ANOVA did not reveal any significant differences between groups in the participants' acoustic measures (Table 9.5). The MFF and SD F° results were analysed using a two-way ANOVA for group and gender. There was a significant difference between diagnostic groups (F = 5.329, p = .021) but no significant difference with post hoc testing. Females had higher MFF values than males (F = 397.294, p < .001), but there was no interaction effect between gender and diagnostic group (F = .158, p = .924). SD F° values are also reported in Table 9.5. There was no significant difference between diagnostic groups (F = .875, p = .549). There was no gender effect (F = .153, p = .719) and no interaction effect between gender and participant group (F = .643, p = .589).

Table 9.4: Percentage of abnormal pre-operative acoustic measures in each diagnostic subgroup

Measure	MNG (n = 48) % abnormal	Cancer (n = 16) % abnormal	Thyro-toxicity (n = 6) % abnormal	Nodule (n = 27) % abnormal	Para-thyroid (n = 15) % abnormal
MPT	42	31	67	48	40
MFF male	25	29	No data	7	17
MFF female	40	19	17	11	33
SD F°	77	56	100	70	60
Jitter	71	75	100	63	47
HNR	50	44	50	48	53
PFR	56	63	50	67	60

Note. MNG = multinodular goitre, MPT = maximum phonation time, SD = standard deviation, MFF = mean fundamental frequency, SD F° = standard deviation of fundamental frequency, HNR = harmonics-to-noise ratio, PFR = phonation frequency range.

Table 9.6 details the percentage of electroglottographic results that were classified as abnormal for participants grouped diagnostically. Normal values for duration of closed phase of cycle (Qx) were considered to be between 40–50% and normal values for irregularity of fundamental frequency (CFx) were considered to be less than 20%. A higher CFx value indicates less regular vocal fold vibration and correlates perceptually with poorer voice quality. Qx indicates the phase during the vocal fold vibratory cycle where the vocal folds close, the maximum contact and the opening phase, but excludes the phase where the vocal folds are fully open (Carlson & Miller 1998).

Table 9.5: Pre-operative acoustic measures by diagnosis

Measures	MNG (n = 48) M (SD)	Cancer (n = 16) M (SD)	Toxicity (n = 6) M (SD)	Nodule (n = 27) M (SD)	Para-thyroid (n = 15) M (SD)	F Value	P value
MPT	11.4 (5)	11.9 (5)	7.8 (2)	11.5 (5)	11.3 (5)	.578	.723
MFF male *	120.5 (21.7)	137.3 (63)	No data	124.3 (36)	122.9 (17.9)		
MFF female *	189.3 (38.7)	221.9 (37)	195.2 (43.5)	205.5 (34)	194 (26.4)		
SD F° *	26 (18)	27.2 (43)	28.5 (13)	23.9 (25)	17 (15)		
Jitter	2.1 (2)	2.5 (5)	2.7 (2)	3 (5)	1.2 (1)	.806	.524
HNR	17.8 (6)	16.4 (7)	15.4 (7)	18.8 (10)	18.5 (5)	.741	.493
PFR	12.8 (5)	12.5 (5)	12.2 (7)	11.7 (5)	13.7 (6)	.383	.820

Note. * Analysed by two-way ANOVA. MNG = multinodular goitre, SD = standard deviation, MFF = mean fundamental frequency, SD F° = standard deviation of fundamental frequency, HNR = harmonics-to-noise ratio, PFR = phonation frequency range.

Table 9.6: Percentage of diagnostic sub-groups with abnormal pre-operative electroglottographic measures

Values	MNG (n = 48) % abnormal	Cancer (n = 16) % abnormal	Toxicity (n = 5) % abnormal	Nodule (n = 27) % abnormal	Para-thyroid (n = 15) % abnormal
Qx	77	56	83	81	80
CFx	50	43	33	63	44

Note. MNG = multinodular goitre, Qx = duration of closed phase cycle of vocal fold vibration, CFx = irregularity of fundamental frequency.

Pre-operative electroglottographic data were statistically analysed using a one-way ANOVA and it was found that there were no significant differences between groups when analysing duration of closed phase cycle of vocal fold vibration (Qx) and irregularity of fundamental frequency (Cfx) (Table 9.7). These are both measures taken in connected speech and have been proposed to correlate with perceptual voice quality (Fourcin 2000). For example, perceptual breathy voice quality is related to a longer open phase, falsetto voice quality corresponds to less rapid vocal fold closure giving a relative lack of higher spectral components (Fourcin 2000).

Table 9.7: Pre-operative electroglottgraphic measures by diagnosis

Values	MNG (n = 48) M (SD)	Cancer (n = 16) M (SD)	Toxicity (n = 5) M (SD)	Nodule (n = 27) M (SD)	Para-thyroid (n = 15) M (SD)	F value	P value
Qx	44 (14)	43.6 (11)	49.5 (15)	42.1 (14)	47.9 (12)	.786	0.537
CFx	30.1 (23)	24.6 (19)	20 (10)	28.3 (20)	22.4 (13)	.526	0.803

Note. M = mean; SD = standard deviation, Qx = duration of closed phase cycle of vocal fold vibration, CFx = irregularity of fundamental frequency.

Table 9.8 displays pre-operative symptom rating scores with participants grouped according to compression status. Participants with definite compression had significantly worse total symptom scores (p = 0.009). Participants with definite compression had more abnormal breathing, cough, voice and upper airway scores (p < .001) than those who did not have compression. Seventy-eight percent of participants with definite compression had abnormal total symptom scores compared to 21% of participants who did not have compression. Specifically, upper airway symptom scores were abnormal in 71% of participants with compression compared to 23% of participants who did not have compression. MFF and SD F° results were analysed using a two-way ANOVA for compression group and gender. Females had significantly higher MFF than males (F = 22.026, p = .001). There was no significant difference between compression groups (F = .156, p = .865), and no interaction effect between gender and compression group (F = 1.460, p = .237). There was no significant difference in SD F° results between compression groups (F = .2953, p = .253) or gender (F = .003, p = .959) and no interaction effect between gender and participant group (F = .493, p = .612).

Table 9.8: Pre-operative symptom scores grouped by compressive status

Symptom score	Compression Present (n = 50) M (SD)	Compression Absent (n = 62) M (SD)	T value	P value
Total	24.0 (15.9)	8.9 (10.7)	5.989	< .001
Breathing	3.9 (3.9)	1.7 (2.4)	3.724	< .001
Cough	5.8 (3.9)	2.2 (2.7)	5.827	< .001
Voice	5.2 (4.9)	2.0 (4.1)	3.847	< .001
Upper airway	9.5 (6.7)	3.7 (4.6)	5.366	< .001

Note. M = mean, SD = standard deviation

Pre-operative acoustic measures grouped by compression status are detailed in Table 9.9. Comparison of acoustic voice measures revealed no significant difference between groups.

There was a significant difference between compressive groups for CFx but not for Qx2 (Table 9.10). Patients with definite compression had more abnormal CFx scores than those with no compression.

Auditory perceptual evaluation of pitch was abnormal in 27% of participants. Less than 1% of all participants had severe pitch abnormality. Five percent of participants were rated as having a moderate pitch abnormality, 8% were rated with a mild pitch abnormality and 13% had a slight pitch abnormality. The remaining 73% of participants were perceived to have normal pitch at their pre-operative voice assessment. The most frequently detected pitch abnormality was low pitch (11%), followed by monopitch (9%) and the least frequently detected pitch abnormality was high pitch (7%).

Table 9.9: Pre-operative acoustic measures grouped by compressive status

Instrumental	Compression present (n = 45) M (SD)	No compression (n = 62) M (SD	T value	P value
MPT	10.9 (4.7)	11.6 (4.8)	−.749	0.455
MFF male	129.6 (33.9)	124.15 (40.2)		
MFF female	186.9 (36.6)	204.3 (35.4)		
SD F°	24.6 (18.8)	24.7 (28.0)		
Jitter	2.7 (3.9)	2.0 (2.7)	1.045	.299
HNR	17.6 (6.3)	18.0 (7.7)	−.316	.752
PFR	12.1 (5.3)	13.0 (5.3)	−.844	.400

Note. M = mean, SD = standard deviation, MFF = mean fundamental frequency, SD F° = standard deviation of fundamental frequency, HNR = harmonics-to-noise ratio, PFR = phonation frequency range

Table 9.10: Pre-operative electroglottographic values grouped by compression

Values	Definite compression (n = 45) M (SD)	No compression (n = 62) M (SD)	T Value	P Value
Qx2	41.9 (13.6)	46.3 (12.3)	−1.758	0.082
CFx	31.8 (24.5)	23.5 (14.7)	2.206	0.030*

Note. M = mean, SD = standard deviation, Qx = duration of closed phase cycle of vocal fold vibration, CFx = irregularity of fundamental frequency, * = significantly different

Eighty-five percent of all participants were rated as having abnormal voice quality at their pre-operative voice assessment appointments. Four percent of participants had a severe quality abnormality, 3% had a moderate–severe quality abnormality, 18% had a moderate quality abnormality, 33% of participants had a mild quality abnormality and 27% of participants had a slight quality abnormality. The remaining 15% were perceived to have normal quality at their pre-operative voice assessment. The most frequently detected quality abnormality was roughness (61%) which correlates with previous reports in the literature of voice change related to malfunction of the thyroid gland. There was strain detected in 59% of participants, breathiness in 41% of participants and glottal fry in 30% of all participants. Additional quality abnormalities less frequently identified pre-operatively were pitch breaks (2%) and diplophonia (1%). An independent t test was used to compare auditory perceptual voice features between compressive groups. For the purpose of this statistical test, patients with possible or early compression were considered to have compression. Abnormal auditory perceptual ratings of pitch were more commonly reported in participants with definite compression ($p = 0.001$), but there was no significant difference of auditory perceptual ratings of quality ($p = .276$) between compression groups. When grouped diagnostically there was no significant difference in perceptual ratings using a one-way ANOVA between groups. For the purposes of this project, loudness was not perceptually rated.

Overall voice results were considered abnormal if they had either: a) a total symptom score outside the normal range, b) one or more moderate, moderate–severe or severe auditory perceptual voice feature, c) three or more abnormal instrumental scores or d) two or more abnormal electroglottographic results. Based on this definition, 80% of participants were classified as having abnormal voice. This suggests that 80% of patients with thyroid disease presented with some abnormality in their voice at their pre-operative voice assessment. Overall, five (4%) participants presented with a clinically significant auditory perceptual abnormality; that is, a rating of *moderate* or above. Thirty-eight (34%) participants had an abnormal total symptom score on the self-reported symptom rating questionnaire. Seventy-four (66%) participants had three or more abnormal instrumental scores such as maximum phonation time (MPT), jitter, harmonic-to-noise ratio etc. Fifty-five (49%) participants had two or more abnormal electroglottographic measures. Only five participants had abnormal results across all domains of testing, i.e. auditory perceptual rating, self-reported symptom rating, acoustic assessment and electroglottography.

Discussion

This research demonstrates a high prevalence of different abnormal voice features in patients referred for pre-operative voice assessment. The results demonstrate that comprehensive speech pathology pre-operative assessment is warranted in this clinical population.

Many text books on voice production and treatment simply report the existence of abnormal features of voice in thyroid disease (Colton et al. 2006; Verdolini et al. 2006). This CDM study identifies various abnormal symptoms, auditory perceptual and instrumental features of participants with various thyroid diseases and parathyroidism.

The results also indicate that, if compression is caused by the thyroid gland, there may be more significant symptoms related to breathing, cough and upper airway problems. Patients with compressive thyroid disease also have more abnormalities in their auditory perceptual voice features than those with no compression. It should be noted, however, that this research only studied patients undergoing surgery for their thyroid disease. Patients whose thyroid disease was managed through medication were not included in the study. Therefore, these results cannot be generalised to the entire population of individuals with thyroid disease.

At this point, we may again ask whether the concept or label of *thyroid voice* is valid. From our results it does not seem plausible that a patient who has thyroid disease severe enough to warrant surgery will present with a specific set of empirically identifiable abnormal vocal features, which are differentiated by disease type. Therefore, we suggest that the label of 'thyroid voice' should not be used. Although voice problems were prevalent, there was not a single set of unique features. We must be wary of assuming that patients with thyroid disease will all manifest with a specific type of voice abnormality.

Prior to the conduct of this CDM study, it was assumed that patients with parathyroid disease rarely had abnormal voice features or reported vocal symptoms. This study demonstrates that patients undergoing parathyroidectomy also had a high prevalence of abnormal vocal features. Therefore, patients undergoing parathyroidectomy also require pre-operative voice assessment as well as monitoring after surgery. The findings of this CDM study have significantly altered the clinical management of thyroid and parathyroid disease patients in our facility. Prior to the study, the speech pathology department considered excluding the latter group of patients from requiring pre- and post-operative voice assessments. Based on the analysis of available empirical data however, parathyroid surgical patients are routinely assessed pre-operatively and some of these have even required voice therapy following surgery.

The results from this study are applicable to the ongoing clinical caseload within the Speech Pathology Department at John Hunter Hospital and could also be applied to similar speech pathology clinics that work with voice and thyroid surgery patients across the world. Pre-operative voice analysis of patients undergoing thyroid or parathyroid surgery is recommended. This testing should be performed by a qualified speech pathologist and should include a multidimensional profile of the patient's voice including patient's self-reported symptoms, auditory perceptual voice analysis, and instrumental assessment. A pre-operative voice assessment clinic is beneficial because concerns about voice from patient, otolaryngologist or speech pathologist can be addressed promptly. By having a clinic available specifically for the surgical voice caseload, including patients with thyroid disease, and maintaining good relationships between the otolaryngologist and speech pathologists, referrals can be processed quickly and it is logistically easier to organise therapy after surgery. Additionally, if patients require further follow-up, the speech pathologist can re-refer to the otolaryngologist.

Limitations

Analysis of data concerning post-operative voice changes in this sample were beyond the scope of this particular study. However, it would be clinically useful to compare the pre-operative features of the voice in patients with thyroid disease to their post-operative vocal features and to identify the change to the voice that occurs following surgery. Post-operative voice data is considered important because patients with thyroid disease are often more concerned by how their voice will change following surgery rather than what it is like pre-operatively.

Another limitation of this study is the large standard deviations for the acoustic measures. There was a large variability in acoustic measures within each diagnostic category. Perhaps this is a function of the extent of disease process. For example, one person with thyroid cancer may have quite invasive disease process extending beyond the thyroid gland itself, interfering with the laryngeal nerves, whereas another individual with thyroid cancer may have a smaller lesion with no effect on voice production at all.

Although clinical information about laryngeal pathology, extent of disease and smoking history is recorded in the hospital medical record, this information was not included in the database and therefore did not form part of the analysis. It is therefore possible that some of these extraneous variables could have impacted on the results. However, anecdotally, the treating clinicians did not believe these factors were prevalent.

Although a few patients did not attend a pre-operative appointment (3%), they represented a small enough subset to not raise question about our findings. Nonetheless, missing data can be equally as instructive in research as data collected and may offer clinically significant 'findings' (Epstein 2010).

Using CDM methodology provides a rich source of 'real world' clinical information. CDM is non-invasive to the patient and does not exclude participants because it gives a sample of all the people who presented to the clinic over a certain time frame. This helps capture a good representation of what to expect of a particular clinical caseload. This in turn means that the results can easily be applied to ongoing clinical practices for that client population.

Conclusions

The authors believe that this empirically based CDM study has significantly improved the clinical care for patients with thyroid disease at the John Hunter Hospital. It is important to explain to pre-operative patients with thyroid disease why their voice may sound abnormal and how their voice may improve, deteriorate, or remain the same post-surgery. Experience working with this caseload has shown that the patients who arrive at the voice clinic pre-operatively are keen to know what the specific outcome will be for them after they undergo surgery on their thyroid gland. This question cannot be answered until we know what the pre-operative status of voice in thyroid disease is and the extent to which factors such as diagnostic subgroup and compression affect voice.

What we have learnt from the process and outcomes of our research to date is of great clinical relevance. This study shows that 80% of people with thyroid disease requiring surgery presented with abnormal vocal features pre-operatively. These voice features were present in all diagnostic groups. Patients with compressive thyroid disease had more abnormal symptoms related to breathing, cough and upper airway difficulties and more abnormal auditory perceptual features compared to people with thyroid disease without compression.

This study was unable to validate the concept of a singular and typical thyroid voice. Thyroid disease encompasses a number of diagnoses within this broad category which may manifest as specific symptoms for each patient. Generally, thyroid disease impacts on vocal function and upper airway symptoms. But to say there is a specific set of symptoms or vocal features for all types of thyroid disease cannot be supported by the current data.

This project has highlighted the need for two additional projects which are currently in the process of analysis. Specifically, we would like to investigate auditory perceptual vocal features of patients with thyroid disease in greater detail. Secondly, we plan to examine voice outcomes for patients undergoing thyroid surgery.

The CDM process that was employed in this study hopefully will encourage clinicians to recognise how data can be obtained from regular clinical populations seen by allied health and medical practitioners. Setting up a data collection process for clinical populations can provide a wealth of information for analysis at a later stage and can assist in the development of quality improvement or other research studies. The process of CDM for patients with thyroid disease, such as the exercise reviewed in this chapter, has shown to be a very valuable and easily applicable research tool in the healthcare environment. It was time-effective to save the patient's voice samples and enter the patient's test results onto a central database such as Microsoft Excel following their assessment. This process shows that practice-based research (PBR) can be a part of every clinician's workload. Accurate and organised data collection as part of clinical workload can support the development of efficient research practice and the development of knowledge, as well as quality improvement within that clinical area.

References

Aronson AE & Bless DM (2009). *Clinical voice disorders.* 4th edn. New York: Thieme Medical Publishers Inc.

Baken RJ & Orlikoff RF (2000). *Clinical measurement of speech and voice.* 2nd edn. San Diego, California: Singular Publishing.

Baker J (2008). The role of psychogenic and psychosocial factors in the development of functional voice disorders. *International Journal of Speech-Language Pathology,* 10(4): 210–30.

Boersma P (2005). PRAAT acoustics program. [Online]. Available: www.fon.hum. uva.nl/praat/manual/Harmonicity.html [Accessed 13 December 2010].

Carlson E & Miller D (1998). Aspects of voice quality: display, measurement and therapy. *International Journal of Language and Communication Disorders,* 33(Supplement): 304–09.

Colton R, Casper J & Leonard R (2006). *Understanding voice problems: a physiological perspective for diagnosis and treatment.* Sydney: Lippincott Williams & Wilkins.

Darley F, Aronson A & Brown J (1975). *Motor speech disorders.* Philadelphia: WB Saunders.

Debruyne F, Ostyn F, Delaere P & Wellens W (1997). Acoustic analysis of the speaking voice after thyroidectomy. *Journal of Voice,* 11(4): 479–82.

Dejonckere PH, Bradley P, Clemente P, Cornut G, Crevier-Buchman L, Van De Heyning P, Remacle M & Woisard V (2001). A basic protocol for functional assessment of voice pathology, especially for investigating the efficacy of (phonosurgical) treatments and evaluating new assessment techniques: guideline elaborated on by the Committee on Phoniatrics of the European Laryngological Society. *European Archives of Oto-Rhino-Laryngology,* 258(2): 77–82.

Epstein I (2010). *Clinical data-mining: integrating practice and research.* New York: Oxford University Press.

Fairbanks G (1960). *Voice and articulation drillbook.* 2nd edn. New York: Harper & Row.

Farrag TY, Samlan RA, Lin FR & Tufano RP (2006). The utility of evaluating true vocal fold motion before thyroid surgery. *The Laryngoscope,* 116: 235–38.

Fourcin A (2000). Voice quality and electroglottography. In R Kent & M Ball (Eds). *Voice quality measurement* (pp285–306). San Diego, CA: Singular Publishing.

Gorham-Rowan M (2004). Acoustic measures of vocal stability during different speech tasks in young women using oral contraceptives: a retrospective study. *The European Journal of Contraception and Reproductive Health Care,* 9(3): 166–72.

Hirano M (1981). *Clinical examination of voice.* Vienna: Springer-Verlag.

Hirano M, Koike Y & Leden HV (1968). Maximum phonation time and air usage during phonation. *Folia Phoniatrica,* 20: 185.

Hong KH & Kim YK (1997). Phonatory characteristics of patients undergoing thyroidectomy without laryngeal nerve injury. *Otolaryngology, Head and Neck Surgery,* 117(4): 399–404.

Koçak S, Aydıntug S, Özbaş S, Koçak I, Küçük B & Baskan S (1999). Evaluation of vocal cord function after thyroid surgery. *European Journal of Surgery,* 165: 183–86.

Koschkee DL & Rammage L (1997). *Voice care in the medical setting.* San Diego, California: Singular Publishing.

McIvor NP, Flint DJ, Gillibrand J & Morton RP (2000). Thyroid surgery and voice-related outcomes. *Australian and New Zealand Journal of Surgery,* 70: 179–83.

Meek P, Carding N, Howard DH & Lennard WJ (2008). Voice change following thyroid and parathyroid surgery. *Journal of Voice,* 22(6): 765–72.

Oates J & Russell A (1998). Learning voice analysis using an interactive multi-media package: development and preliminary evaluation. *Journal of Voice,* 12(4): 500–12.

Ortega J, Cassinello N, Dorcaratto D & Leopaldi E (2009). Computerized acoustic voice analysis and subjective scaled evaluation of the voice can avoid the need for laryngoscopy after thyroid surgery. *Surgery,* 145(3): 265–71.

Sataloff RT, Emerich KA & Hoover CA (1997). Endocrine dysfunction. In R Sataloff (Ed). *Professional voice: the science and art of clinical care* (pp291-97). 2nd edn. San Diego, CA: Singular Publishing.

Soylu L, Ozbas S, Uslu H Y & Kocak S (2007). The evaluation of the causes of subjective voice disturbances after thyroid surgery. *The American Journal of Surgery,* 194: 317–22.

Speyer R, Wieneke GH & Dejonckere PH (2004). Documentation of progress in voice therapy: perceptual, acoustic and laryngostroboscopic findings pretherapy and posttherapy. *Journal of Voice,* 18(3): 325–40.

Stassen H, Kuny S & Bomben G (2005). Normative study of 192 healthy volunteers. [Online]. Available: www.bli.uzh.ch/vox03.html [Accessed 28 April 2011].

Stojadinovic A, Shaha A, Orlikoff RF, Nissan A, Kornak MF, Singh B, Boyle JO, Shah JP, Brennan MF & Kraus DH (2002). Prospective functional voice assessment in patients undergoing thyroid surgery. *Annals of Surgery*, 236(6): 823–32.

The Speech Pathology Association of Australia Limited (2010). What is a speech pathologist? Fact Sheet 1.1. [Online]. Available: www.speechpathologyaustralia. org.au/library/1.1_What_is_a_Speech_Pathologist.pdf [Accessed 27 January 2011].

Tortora GJ & Derrickson B (2007). The endocrine system. In G J Tortora & B Derrickson (Eds). *Introduction to the human body: essentials of anatomy and physiology* (pp323–25). 7th edn. New York: John Wiley & Sons.

Verdolini K, Rosen CA & Branski RC (2006). *Classification manual for voice disorders–I*. New Jersey: Lawrence Erlbaum Associates.

Vertigan AE, Theodoros DG, Gibson PG & Winkworth AL (2007). Voice and upper airway symptoms in people with chronic cough and paradoxical vocal fold movement. *Journal of Voice*, 21(3): 361–83.

Vertigan AE, Theodoros DG, Winkworth AL & Gibson PG (2008). Acoustic and electroglottographic features of chronic cough and paradoxical vocal fold movement. *Folia Phoniatrica et Logopaedica*, 60: 210–16.

Whybrow PC & Bauer M (2005). Behavioural and psychiatric aspects of thyrotoxicosis. In LE Braverman & RD Utiger (Eds). *Werner & Ingbar's the thyroid: a fundamental and clinical textbook* (pp644–50). Philadelphia, Pennsylvania: Lippincott, Williams & Wilkins.

Acronyms

ADL	activities of daily living
AHMIS	Allied Health Management Information System
AHPA	Allied Health Professions Australia
ANOVA	Analysis of Variance between groups
AR-DRG	Australian refined – diagnostic related group
AusTOMS	Australian Therapy Outcome Measures
BDH	Belmont District Hospital
BEST-2	Bedside Evaluation Screening Test for Aphasia – 2
CBT	cognitive behavioural therapy
CDH	Cessnock District Hospital
CDM	Clinical data mining
CFx	irregularity of fundamental frequency
CHIME	Community Health Information Management Exchange
CINAHL	Cumulative Index to Nursing and Allied Health Literature
CMN	Calvary Mater Newcastle
COT	Client Outcomes Tool
CQx	irregularity of closed phase cycle of vibration
DRG	Diagnostic Related Groups
DSM-IV	*Diagnostic and statistical manual of mental disorders – 4th edition*
DSP	Disability Support Pension
ED	Emergency Department
EBP	evidence-based practice
EPA	electrophysical agents
FASF	forearm support frame

GCS	Glasgow Coma Scale
GHQ	General Health Questionnaire
GNAHN	Greater Newcastle Acute Hospital Network
HADS	Hospital Anxiety and Depression Scale
HCV	hepatitis C virus
HIE	Health Information Exchange
HNE	Hunter New England Health
HNR	harmonics-to-noise ratio
HRT	Health Round Table
ICD	International Classification of Diseases
ICD-9	International Classification of Diseases – 9
ICD-10-CM	International Classification of Diseases-10-Clinical Modification
ICD-10-PCS	International Classification of Diseases-10-Procedure Coding System
ICF	International Classification of Function
IDU	injecting drug use
IFI	Indicators for Intervention
IFN	Interferon
ILU	independent living unit
IQR	interquartile range
IVD	intervertebral disc
JHH	John Hunter Hospital
LAC	Lacunar Stroke
LBP	low back pain
LOS	length of stay
L/S	lumbar spine
M	mean
MBS	Medical Benefits Scheme
MCID	minimum clinically important difference
MFF	mean fundamental frequency
MMSE	Mini Mental Status Examination
MNG	multinodular goitre
MPT	maximum phonation time
NAHBC	National Allied Health Benchmarking Consortium
NAHCC	National Allied Health Casemix Committee

NEWCAT	Newcastle University's Library Catalogue
NHMRC	National Health and Medical Research Council
NSLBP	non-specific low back pain
OOS	occasions of service
PAC	Partial Anterior Circulation Stroke
PBR	practice-based research
PCS	Petersen Classification System
Peg-IFN	pegylated (long-acting) Interferon
PFR	Phonation frequency range
PGI	Patient Generated Index
PLS	Psychiatry Liaison Service
POC	Posterior Circulation Stroke
PSFS	Patient Specific Functional Scale
QA	quality assurance
Qx	duration of closed phase cycle of vocal fold vibration
RBP	research-based practice
RBV	Ribavirin
RCT	randomised control trial
RHSP	Rural Hunter Service Provider (Network)
RM-18	Roland-Morris Disability Questionnaire – 18
RNC	Royal Newcastle Centre
SAH	Sub Arachnoid Haemorrhage
SARRAH	Services for Australian Rural and Remote Allied Health
SD	standard deviation
SDH	Sub Dural Haemorrhage
SD F°	standard deviation of fundamental frequency
SPSS	Statistical Package for the Social Sciences
SRS	Session Ratings Scale
STI	soft tissue injury
TAC	Total Anterior Circulation Stroke
TBI	traumatic brain injury
TKR	total knee replacement
WNL	within normal limits
WPTAS	Westmead Post Traumatic Amnesia Scale

Index

www.ingramcontent.com/pod-product-compliance
Lightning Source LLC
Chambersburg PA
CBHW070349200326
41518CB00012B/2183